Henry Salim Siregar

L-Selectin P213S Polymorphism and Macrophage Profiles in Endometriosis

AF153308

Henry Salim Siregar

L-Selectin P213S Polymorphism and Macrophage Profiles in Endometriosis

An New Insight into the Pathophysiology of Endometriosis

LAP LAMBERT Academic Publishing

Imprint

Any brand names and product names mentioned in this book are subject to trademark, brand or patent protection and are trademarks or registered trademarks of their respective holders. The use of brand names, product names, common names, trade names, product descriptions etc. even without a particular marking in this work is in no way to be construed to mean that such names may be regarded as unrestricted in respect of trademark and brand protection legislation and could thus be used by anyone.

Cover image: www.ingimage.com

Publisher:
LAP LAMBERT Academic Publishing
is a trademark of
Dodo Books Indian Ocean Ltd. and OmniScriptum S.R.L publishing group

120 High Road, East Finchley, London, N2 9ED, United Kingdom
Str. Armeneasca 28/1, office 1, Chisinau MD-2012, Republic of Moldova, Europe
Managing Directors: Ieva Konstantinova, Victoria Ursu
info@omniscriptum.com

Printed at: see last page
ISBN: 978-3-659-63551-9

Zugl. / Approved by: Medan, University of Sumatra Utara, 2014

Table of Contents

Chapter 1
Introduction

Endometriosis is a benign disease defined as an extra uterine presence of endometrial glands and stromas, and is associated with pelvic pain and infertility. Clinical manifestations are usually broad spectrum and highly progressive and with high recurrence rates, and frequently cause treatment complicating issues for both patients and clinicians (Fritz et al., 2011). 10% of reproductive aged women, of all ethnic and social groups, are diagnosed with this disease (Eskenazi et al., 2011). Approximately 20-40% infertile women are diagnosed with endometriosis (Strathy et al., 1982; Verkauf et al., 1987).

Endometriosis causes serious physical, mental, and social implications (Jones et al., 2004; Lorencatto et al., 2006) and is also an economic burden to the society. Simoens et al estimated a US national cost of approximately 22 billion USD in 2002 (Simoens et al., 2007). Hummelshoj et al reported that 78% of women diagnosed with endometriosis in UK lost an average of 5,3 working days due to this disease (Hummelshoj et al., 2006).

However, the pathogenesis is not fully understood (Baziad et al., 2008). A theory by Sampson in the mid 20s was unable to explain as to why endometriosis only occurs on a few amount of women. Most women experience retrograde menstruation (76-90%) that flows into the peritoneal cavity, however, endometriosis is only evident in 5-10% of these cases (Bulun et al., 2009). Therefore, endometriosis may not only involve retrograde menstruation but also other factors on the molecular level, including genetic defects and immune system or both, eg. endometrial cell adhesion and invasion, proliferation, angiogenesis, and immune system dettachment (Sundqvist et al., 2011).

Endometriosis has several genetic predispositions (Fritz et al., 2011). Several data indicate that endometriosis is associated with subclinical peritoneal inflammation characterized by increased peritoneal volume, peritoneal white blood cell concentration (especially increased macrophage activities), and increased inflammatory cytokinees, growth factors, and angiogenic supporting substances (D'Hooghe et al., 2007).

Due to potencial T cell regulatory changes, T cells, B cells, mast and dendritic cell and macrophages are altered, from which ectopic lesions may occur, affecting the events of endometriosis and its progresivisity (Berbic et al., 2011). Several studies have shown altered immune cell function in endometriosis women, indicated by decreased cytoyoxic T cell and Natural killer cell activities, cytokinee secretion by T cell helpers, and autoantibody production by lymphocyte B (Osuga et al., 2011).

Macrophages are normally located in the peritoneum, the amount and activities of which are markedly increased in endometriosis women (Fritz et al., 2011). A study on rats indicated that alternatively activated macophages (M2) dramatically increased growth of endometriosis lesions, whereas inflammatory macrophages (M1) effectively protected them from endometriosis (Bacci et al., 2009).

L-selectin functions in the initital recruitment of circulating leukocytes in to peripheral inflammatory sites, known as rolling leukocytes followed, by activation, of marked adhesion, and leukocyte transmigration to interstitial tissues (Hafezi et al., 2001).

A immunohistochemical study comparing L-selectin locations in rat model endometriosis tissues and human counterparts revealed that L-selectin was more dominantly expressed in interstitial spaces, including macrophages and lymphocytes compared to endometriosis epithelium, and concluded that L-selectin plays a significant role in the pathogenesis of endometriosis (Odagiri et al., 2007).

No study has previously assessed the association between L-selectin gene Polymorphism with endometriosis. This study was therefore conducted to assess the association between P213S polymorphism with events of endometriosis, and to observe the role of alternatively activated macrophages (M2) compared to scavenger macrophages (M1) in the pathogenesis of this disease.

Chapter 2
Literature Review

Definition

Endometriosis is a benign disease defined by the presence of extra uterine ectopic endometrial glands and stromas and is associated with pelvic pain and infertility. This disease has an extensive spectrum of clinical manifestations that tend to progress and recur, and frequently causes complications, both clinically and medically. Although the pathogenesis is not fully understood, a new insight obtained from recent studies using genetic, molecular, and biochemical methods has helped us to better understand the mechanism underlying this disease together with the clinical consequences, and has thus provided a new approach in diagnosing and treating this complex disorder (Fritz et al., 2011).

Epidemiology

Endometriosis is frequently encountered in reproductive aged women. Although uncertain, prevalence rates in certain groups have been frequently reported. Endometriosis occur in approximately 10% of reproductive aged women (Eskenazi et al., 1997), of all ethnic and social groups. Approximately 20-40% of women (Strathy et al., 1982, Verkauf, 1987) with infertility are diagnosed with endometriosis. Patients are averagedly aged between 25 to 35 years old when diagnosed with the disease (Kuohung et al., 2002; Hediger et al., 2005). Endometriosis is less frequently reported in premenarche adolescent females but can be identified in more than 50% of women aged under 20 years old complaining chronic pelvic pain or dyspereunia (Chatman et al., 1986; Goldstein et al., 1989; Reese et al., 1996). Surgery is usually mandatory in less than 5% of post menopausal women dominantly treated with estrogen due to endometrisosis. Compared to Caucasian women, prevalence rates of asymptomatic endometriosis is somewhat lower and higher in Negroid and Asian women, respectively (Sangi-Haghpeykar et al., 1995; Missmer et al., 2004;Fritz et al., 2011).

Risk for endometriosis increases in early menache and short menstrual cycled women. However, the correlation reported between the latter and the disease is inconsistent (Cramer et al., 2002). Reported data on primates show that exposure to polychlorinated biphenyl (PCB) or dioxin may be associated with endometriosis, however, another study on this matter revealed inconsistent results (Rier et al., 2003). Other data have shown that inutero exposure may play a role in developing the disease, indicating that incidence rates of prenatal endometriosis increased in diethylstil besterol-exposed women (Missmer , et al., 2004; Fritz et al., 2011).

Endometriosis has a profound effect on a women's pyhical, mental, and social well-being (Jones, et al., 2004, Lorencatto, et al., 2006) and is also a significant issue as reflected upon the consequent economic burden brought to the society. Simoens et al estimates an additional 22 billion US dollar annual spendings in 2002 due to endometriosis (Simoens, et al., 2007). Hummelshoj et al reported that 78% of women diagnosed with endometriosis in UK lost an average of 5,3 working days due to this disease (Hummelshoj, et al., 2006).

Diagnosis

Endometriosis should be suspected in women with subfertility, dysmenorrhea, dyspareunia, or chronic pelvic pain. However, these symptoms may also be caused by othe diseases. Endometriosis is usually asymptomatic, for instance in several women diagnosed with an advanced stage of the disease (endometrioma or deep infiltrating rectovaginalis endometriosis), whereas women with minimal-mild endometriosis may also present with severe pain (Koninckx et al., 1991; Cornillie et al., 1990; Chapron et al. 2003; Fauconnier et al., 2002; D'Hooghe et al, 2007). Dysmenorrhea is frequently reported; cases of new, progressive, or severe onset would most likely support the possibilities of endometriosis (Mahmood   et al.; Fritz et al., 2011). Several other studies have also shown that inflammatory factors are associated with infertility. L-selectin ligands have shown to effect blastocyst implantation (Margarit et al., 2009).

Physical examination of external genitals usually show normal findings. Inspeculum may occasionally reveal easily bleeding typical blue or red proliferative implants, usually lolated on the posterior fornix. Although rarely observed, endometriosis is frequently palpated in cases of deep infiltrating endometriosis (Fauconnier et al., 2002). A retroversed, fixated or immobile uterus is also a common finding. Fixated adnexal masses may also accompany women with endometriosis. Utero sacral local tenderness and nodularity is usually suggestive for endometriosis and is frequently the only clue observed during physical examination (Ripps et al., 1992; Matorras et al., 1996). Although reported with highest sensitivity values during

4

menstruation, a physical examination may not always exclude endometriosis upon normal findings (Koninckx et al., 1996). Overall, compared to surgery as the gold standard for diagnosis, physical examination has poor sensitivity, specificity, and predictive values (Spaczynski et al., 2003; Fritz et al., 2011).

The presence of filling defects (hypertrophic endometrium and polypoid) detected during a hysterosalphgynographic examination positively correlates with endometriosis. These findings have positive and negative predictive values of 84% and 75%, respectively. Tranvaginal or transrectal sonography is an essential diagnostic tool in assessing ovarian endometriosis cysts (a differentiation of other adnexal masses) and rectovaginal endometriosis (sensitivity and specificity of 97% and 96%, respectively), however it is less effective in assessing pelvic adhesions or superficial peritoneal endometriosis focuses.

Other imaging techniques, including computed tomography (CT) and MRI, may be used to provide additional information and confirmation (differentiating ovarian endometrioma from other ovarian cystic masses). However, as costs are higher, these modailities are usually not employed for primary diagnosis (Bazot et al., 2007; Arrive et al., 1989; Togashi et al., 1991). Superior results for detecting peritoneal implants are usually yielded from MRI tests than transvaginal sonography (Zeitoun et al., Fritz et al, 2011; D'Hooghe et al., 2007).

Currently, no reliable biomarker has been accepted in diagnosing and determining the prognosis of endometriosis. Various serum liquor and peritoneal markers, including cancer antigene 125 (CA-125) and cytokinees, including interleukine (IL-6) abd Tumor Necrosis Factor (TNF)–α, have been proposed. Although yielding promising results, further studies are neccesary to evalauate the diagnostic relevance of these biormarkers (Sundqvist, 2011).

Diagnostic laparoscopy is the main method used to diagnose endometriosis. Laparoscopic findings usually vary and may include a typical endometriosis, endometrioma, and adhesion formations. Pelvic organs and peritonemum are typical locations for endometriosis. Laparoscopic appearance of these lesions vary and may appear reddish, white, and blackish.(Figure 1)

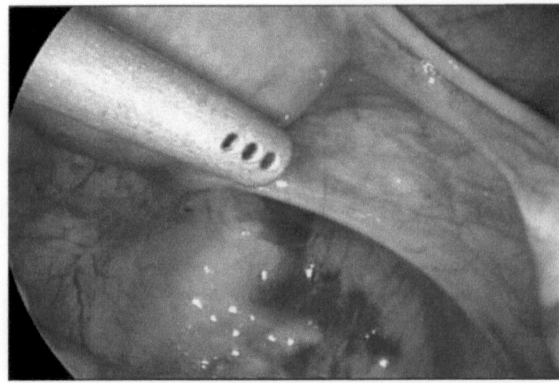

Figure 1. Below the irigator tip, red and white endometriosis lesions are present in the pelvic peritoneum during laparoscopy *(Courtesy of Dr. Karen Bradshaw.)*

Dark lesion are usually pigmented with hemosiderin deposits from entrapped menstrual debris. White and red lesions most frequently correlated with histological findings of endometriosis. Apart from pigmentation, endometriosis lesions also differ morphologically. Endometriosis lesions may also appear as smooth blebs on the peritoneal surface, peritoneal filling defects, or smooth star shaped lesions with points formed by surrouding scar tissues. Lesion may be superficial or deeply infiltrate peritoneal space or pelvic organs (Carr, 2008).

Histopathological confirmation is essential in diagnosing endometriosis. Microscopically, endometriosis implants consist of endometrial glands and stromas with or without homesiderine containing macrophages. Microscopic endometriosis designates the presence of peritoneal endometrial glands and stroma in a macroscopically normal peritoneum. A series of normal laparoscopic biopsies reported that of the total normal peritoneal samples, 10 to 15% of subjects evidently had microscopic endometriosis, with 6% non macroscopic endometriosis patients positively confirmed for the disease (Nisolle et al., 1990; Balasch et al., 1996; Nezhat et al., 1991; D'Hooghe et al., 2007).

Stages of Endometriosis

Staging in endometriosis is essential, especially to determine the appropriate treatment and to evaluate response to medication. Currently, the system used in classifying endometriosis is based on the American Fertility Society (AFS), which is described as follows (Roberts et al., 2003):

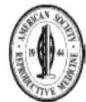

AMERICAN SOCIETY FOR REPRODUCTIVE MEDICINE
REVISED CLASSIFICATION OF ENDOMETRIOSIS

Patient's Name _____ Date _____

Stage I (Minimal) - 1–5	Laparoscopy _____ Laparotomy _____ Photography _____
Stage II (Mild) - 6–15	Recommended treatment _____
Stage III (Moderate) - 16–40	
Stage IV (Severe) - >40	

Total _____ Prognosis _____

PERITONEUM	ENDOMETRIOSIS		< 1 cm	1–3 cm	> 3 cm
	Superficial		1	2	4
	Deep		2	4	6
OVARY	R	Superficial	1	2	4
		Deep	4	16	20
	L	Superficial	1	2	4
		Deep	4	16	20
	POSTERIOR CUL-DE-SAC OBLITERATION		Partial		Complete
			4		40
	ADHESIONS		< 1/3 Enclosure	1/3–2/3 Enclosure	> 2/3 Enclosure
OVARY	R	Filmy	1	2	4
		Dense	4	8	16
	L	Filmy	1	2	4
		Dense	4	8	16
TUBE	R	Filmy	1	2	4
		Dense	4*	8*	16
	L	Filmy	1	2	4
		Dense	4*	8*	16

* If the fimbriated end of the Fallopian tube is completely enclosed, change the point assignment to 16

Denote appearance of superficial implant types as red ([R], red, red–pink, flamelike, vesicular blobs, clear vesicles), white ([W], opacifications, peritoneal defects, yellow–brown) or black ([B], black, hemosiderin deposits, blue). Denote percent of total described as R___% W___% and B___%. Total should equal 100%.

Additional Endometriosis: _____ Associated Pathology: _____

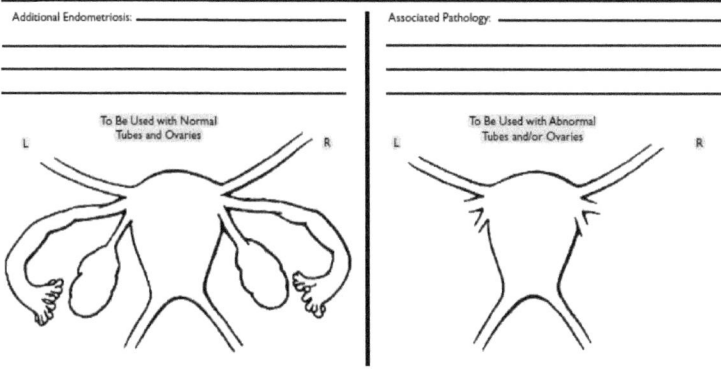

To Be Used with Normal Tubes and Ovaries

To Be Used with Abnormal Tubes and/or Ovaries

Figure 2. Classification of Endometriosis Based on The revised American Society for Reproductive Medicine

Treatment

Treatments include prevention, observation, hormonal therapy, and surgery (Prabowo, 2005).

No unified strategy has been proven succesfull in preventing endometriosis. Protective effects resulting from physical excercises has yet to be fully studied. Facts supporting possible protective effects of oral contraceptive use against the progression of endometriossis are also inadequate (D'Hooghe et al., 2007).

Endometriosis is treated surgically and/or pharmacologically, the treament of which is aimed on: reducing pain, increasing fertility/pregnancy rates and preventing recurrencies. Most pharmacalogical treatments are based on hormonal supression, causing a hypoestrogenic state and elimination or size reduction of endometriosis lesions. Progestin, danazol, gonadotropin-releasing hormone (GnRH) analogues, Levonorgestrel-Releasing Intrauterine System (LNG-IUS) and oral contraseptive use comprises current available pharmacological treatments. Several medications, including LNG-IUS (Mirena) may reduce pain, but apparently has no effect on the disease. Hormonal suppresion using certain medications, including GnRH for a prolonged period of time may cause adverse effects due to systemic estrogen deficiency (Sundqvist, 2011).

Other pharmacological treatments, including Non-Steroidal Anti-Inflammatory Drugs (NSAIDs), are widely used to treat chronic pelvic pain in patients with endometriosis. Regressed lesions in rats have been observed during treatment using aromatase inhibitors (letrozole). Decreased pain has also been observed in human treated with either only aromatase inhibitors or combination with other oral conraceptives (Sundqvist, 2011). Treatment using aromatase inhibtors are indicated in cases showing resistance to standard medication, as not only do they inhibit estrogen production in endometrial tissues, but also inhibit estrogen prodcution in fat and skin tissues. Whereas treatment using selective estrogen receptor modulators (SERM) in rat models with raloxifene therapy, may result in regression of endometriosis (Buelke et al., 1998; D'Hooghe et al., 2007).

Alternative non-hormonal therapies to treat endometriosis have been proposed, including immunomodulators, anti-angiogenic agents and anti-inflammatory drugs. For example, treatment using anti-TNF antibodies have been shown to decrease the extent of endometriosis in baboons (Falconer, et al., 2006; Sundqvist, 2011).

Surgical approach to treat endometriosis is aimed on restoring or recovering normal inter-anatomical association, to excise or disrupt all visible endometriosis lesions, and to pospone recurrences and reduce pain. As pharmacological approaches are ineffective, surgery would be a method of choice for women with moderate to severe endometriosis, a distorted anatomy, and still desiring offsprings (Fritz et al., 2011). Although surgery has proven effective in reducing pain, endometriosis lesion usually recur in several years. Surgery in cases of ovarian endometriosis cysts is associated with decreased ovarian reserve (Sundqvist, 2011).

Surgical procedures are performed laparoscopically or laparotomically. Laparoscopy may be considered in all cases, except cases with difficulties in tissue dissecting or circumstances that neccesitate optimal entry to facilitate atraumatic manipulation of the organs involved. Specific endoscopic procedures comprise of endometriosis implant ablation, adhesiolysis, ovarian cystectomy, oophorectomy, and salphyngectomy (Hesla et al., 2008).

Conservative resection of endometriosis lesions using laparotomical approach is most optimally used in cases of wide spreaded endometriosis, strong pelvic adhesions or endometriomas measuring more than 5 cm. In addition, deep infiltrating endomertriosis involving the rectovaginal septum with fibrosis enhancend to the perirectal fossae, invasion to intestinal tissues, and infiltration through uterine vascular regions and urether in general, is most optimally approached through laparotomy. This latter procedure aims on complete excision of all endometriosis lesions and attachments to restore the functional anatomy of the reproductive tract. Surgical approach is usually performed through a suprapubic transversal inscision. A Maylard Inscision provides adequate exposure for pre saral neurectomy and reconstructive surgery for ovarian endometrioma of almost all sizes (Hesla et al., 2008).

Pathogenesis

The pathogenesis of endometriosis is not fully understood. Several theories have been proposed to explain the histogenesis of endometriosis (Baziad, 2008):

• *The theory of implantantion (Sampson)*, explains that endometriosis occurs due to viable endometrial cells depositing in to the peritoneal cavity by retrograde menstruation, passing through the fallopian tube, resulting in remotely attached and growing endometrial cells.

• *The theory of metaplasia*, stresses an epithilial coelemic (metaplasia) transformation as the basis of endometriosis. The events are insitu in nature, originating from local tissues, including remnants from the Mullerian and Wolffian ducts.

• *The theory of indcution* explains that an abdominal cavity degrading endometrium releases factors, consequently inducing mesenchymal cellular metaplasia that eventually results in endometriosis.

The most widely accepted theory today is the theory of implantation proposed by Sampson in the mid 20s, that provides a logical mechanism for most endometriosis lesions. Unfortunely, this theroy fails to explain the fact that apparently endometriosis only occurs in a small portion of women. Later studies have reported that 76-90% of women experience retrograde menstruation flowing to the peritoneal cavity, however endometriosis was only evident in 5-10% of these cases (Bulun, 2009). Therefore, endometriosis may not only involve retrograde menstruation, but also other factors on the molecular level, including genetic defects, immune system or both, eg. endometrial cell adhesion and invasion, proliferation, angiogenesis, and immune system dettachment. Furthermore, genetic predispositions are apparently involved in the pathogenesis of endometriosis (Matarese et al., 2003; Sundqvist, 2011).

Most facts show that endometriosis is associated with a subclinical peritoneal inflammatory state, characterized by increased peritoneal volume, increased peritoneal leukocyte concentration (especially macrophages with associated increased activities), and increased inflammatory cytokinees, growth factors, and angiogenesis supporting substances (D'Hooghe et al., 2007). Consequently, endometriosis is an inflammatory condition, characterized by marked recruited leukocyte count from the circulating system to endometriosis lesions, resulting in altered eutopic endometrial leukocyte counts, functions and endometriosis lesions. T cell, B cell, mast cell, dendritic cell and macrophages in endometrium and ectopic endometriosis lesions have been shown to undergo alterations, possibly as a result of potential changes in T regulator cells, affecting the occurence and progresivisity of endometriosis (Berbic et al., 2011). Most studies have shown that immune cells undergo functional changes in women with endometriosis, including decreased cytotoxic T cell and NK cell, T cell helper-mediated cytokinee secretion, and B lymphocyte produced by autoantibody activities (Osuga et al., 2011).

Inflamation and Immune Response

Several facts adequately proved that endometriosis is associated with a subclinical peritoneal inflammatory state, characterized by increased peritoneal liquid volume, leukocyte concentration (especially macrophages with increased activities), and increased inflammatory cytokinees, growth factors, and angiogenic supporting substances. Reports on baboons showed that subclinical peritoneal inflamation occured during menstruation and after intrapelvic peritoneal injections (D'Hooge et al., 2006). Higher basal activation rates of peritoneal macrophages in patients with endometriosis may alter fertility by reducing sperm motility and increasing sperm phagocytosis or by increasing cytokinee levels, including TNF-α. TNF-α may also facilitate pelvic endometrial implantation. Endometrial stromal cell attachement to in vitro mesothelial cells could be increased through pretreatment using mesothelial cells with physiological dosages of TNF-α (Zhang et al., 1993). Macrophages may support endometrial cellular grwoth by secreting growth factors and angiogenetic factors, including epidermal growth factors (EGF), macrophage-derived growth factors (MDGF), fibronectin, and adhesion molecules (eg. integrin). On attaching to endometrial cells to the peritoneum, further invasion and growth seem to be regulated by matrix metalloproteinase (MMP) and tissue factor pathway inhibitors (Sillem et al., 1999; Olive et al., 1991; Sharpe et al., 1992; D'Hooghe et al., 2007).

Inflammatory cytokines play a central role in regulating cellular proliferation, motility, adhesion, chemotaxis, and morphogenesis. Several cytokinees, including IL-1, IL-5, IL-6, IL-8, IL-15, monocyte chemotactic protein-1 (MCP-1), TNF-α, transforming growth factor-β (TGF-β) and Regulated on Activation, Normal T-cell Expressed dan Secreted (RANTES) have been implicated in the pathogenesis of endometriosis. Several cytokinee levels have also been observed to be correlated with severity degrees of the disease. TNF-α, IL-8, and MCP-1 have higher expression rates in the early stage of the disease and gradually decrease in advance stages, whereas decreased expressions of TGF-β coincide with severity degrees. RANTES is also increased in peritoneal women diagnosed with more severe degrees of endometriosis (Lebovic et al., 2001; Pizzo et al., 2002; Khorram, et al., 1993; Sundqvist, 2011).

A healthy immune system eliminates ectopic endometrial cells and prevents implantation and progression to endometriosis lesions. This process may be facilitated by changes in endometrial cell apoptosis, that normally increases by the end of the menstrual cycle, however, the process is significantly decreased in cases of endometriosis. Therefore, in healthy women, endometrial cells disseminated to the ectopic location may be programmed to undergo death and is easily eliminated by the immune system. A resulting cellular immune system deficiency or endometrial Z cellular decrease, then occurs, possibly causing inappropriate endometrial survival and cellular implantation (Paul, et al., 2004).

Endometriosis may be a result of decreased peritoneal endometrial cellular washings due to decreased NK cellular activities or decreased macrophage activities. Cellular mediated reduced cytoytoxies on autologous endometrial cells have been associated with endometriosis (D'Hooghe et al., 2007).

Therefore, endometriosis is an inflammatory condition characterized by massive recruitment of leukocytes from the circulating system to endometriosis lesions, consequently resulting in altered leukocyte counts and functions. Macrophages, natural killer cells, and T lymphocytes, B lymphocytes, mast cells, and dendritic cells are increased in endometriosis lesions though extravasation from the circulating system in to endometriosis lesions, from which functions of T regulator cells undergo alterations, consequently affecting occurence and progressivity of endometrioisis (Berbic et al., 2011).

L-selectin functions in the initital recruitment of circulating leukocytes in to peripheral inflammatory sites, known as rolling leukocytes, followed by activation, marked adhesion, and leukocyte transmigration to interstitial tissues (Hafezi Moghadam, et al., 2001). L-selectin is also associated with an implantation process. L-selectin is also known to be more higly expressed in preovulatory phase than proliferating phase. Consequently L-selectin is also frequently associated with events of infertility (Horne et al., 2002; Lai et al., 2005).

A immunohistochemical study comparing L-selectin locations in rat model endometriosis tissues and human counterparts revealed that L-selectin was more dominantly expressed in interstitial spaces, including macrophages and lymphocytes compared to endometriosis epithelium, and concluded that L-selectin plays a significant role in the pathogenesis of endometriosis (Odagiri et al., 2007). Several studies from the Department of Obstetrics and Gynecology, Faculty of Medicine, University of Sumatera Utara, showed significant L-selectin expressions in women with endometriosis tissues compared to non endometriosis tissues. Several other cytokinee associated studies that play a role in endometriosis have also been performed (table 1).

Table 1. Results of studies conducted at the Department of Obstetrics and Gynecology, Faculty of Medicine, University of Sumatera Utara

L-Selectin expression in endometriosis tissues compared to non-endometriosis lesions	Significant difference with p< 0,0001.	Nasution et al., 2014
sL-selectin levels in endometriosis compared to non endometriosis tissues	Endometriosis sL-Selectin mean value of 1018,1(191,7) ng/ml. Non-endometriosis sL-Selectin mean value of 985,6 (195,2) ng/ml with p=0,47	Marpaung et al., 2014
Immunohistochemical expression of aromatase p450 in ectopic endometrium of endometriosis subjects compared to the normal endometrium	Significant difference with p<0,0001	Manurung et al., 2014
Matrix metalloproteinase-9 (MMP-9) expressions in endometriosis tissues than endometrium	Significant difference with p<0,0001	Sembiring et al., 2014
Endometriosis VEGF serum levels compared to endometriosis	Endometriosis VEGF mean levels: 436,64±176,87	Fahmi et al., 2014

13

subjects	Non-Endometriosis 182,22±57,23 with p < 0,0001	
IL-2 values in women with endometriosis and non endometriosis subjects	Endometriosis Mean IL-2 values : 6,3±2,6 Non-Endometriosis Mean IL-2 values : 36,8±10,8 with p < 0,0001	Darya et al., 2014
IL-6 levels in endometriosis and non endometriosis subjects	Endometriosis Mean IL-6 values: 13,1±7,4 Non-Endometriosis 2,2±1,5 with p < 0,0001	Saputra et al., 2014

Role of l-selectin in Leukocyte Extravasation
Selectin structure

Selectin is a family originated from three cellular surface type-I glycoproteins, including E-, L-, and P-selectin. L-selectin is expressed in all granulocytes, monocytes and most lymphocytes. P-selectin is stored in α-granules, originated from platelets and endothelial Weibel-Palade bodies. E-selectin is not regularly expressed (apart from dermal micro vasculars), but it could be immediately induced by other inflammatory cytokines (Klaus L, 2003).

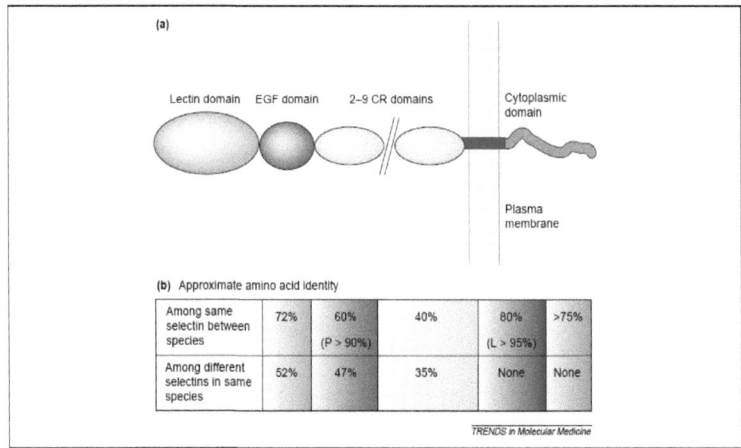

(a)

Lectin domain   EGF domain   2–9 CR domains   Cytoplasmic domain

Plasma membrane

(b) Approximate amino acid identity

Among same selectin between species	72%	60% (P > 90%)	40%	80% (L > 95%)	>75%
Among different selectins in same species	52%	47%	35%	None	None

Figure 3. Selectin structures (a). Selectin comprises of N-terminal lectin domains (bright green), and epidermal growth factor (EGF) domain (dark green), two (L-Selectin), six (E-Selectin) or nine (P-Selectin) consensus repeat with homology to complement regulatory (CR) proteins (yellow), a domain transmembrane domain (red) and cytoplasmic domain (violet) (b). Identity sequwnce of amino acids in each domain between various spesies (human, rat, and bovine) and between three Selectin types in the same spesies (Ley, 2003)

Selectins apparently have significant sequence homologous levels between the three selectin types encountered in the species (apart from the transmembran and cytoplasmic domain) and between each species. Analysis on this matter revealed that lectin domain (binding glucose clusters) is the most preserved domain, thus stating that the three selectin types bind similar glucose clusters. Intrestingly, cytoplasmic and transmembran domains are the most preserved domains between species, however, this does not apply to selectins. These various selectin molecular parts are responsible for each different compartment: P-selectin for secreting granules, E-selectin for membrane plasma, and L-Selectin for leukocyte micro fold ends (Klaus L, 2003).

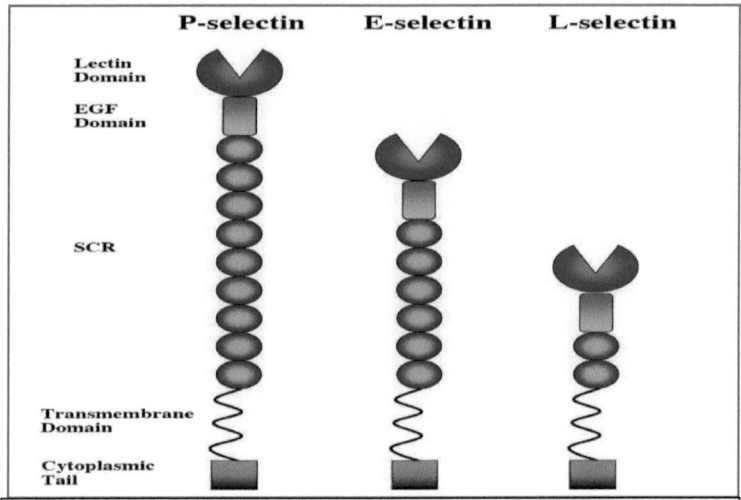

Figure 4. P, E, and L-Selectin structures. Selectin consists of binding lectin domain, domains such as epidermal growth factors (EGF), a series of short consensus repeats (SCR), and transmembran domain and cytomplasmic tail. P-Selectin has 9 SCRs, E-selectin has 6 SCRs, and L-Selectin has 2 SCRs (Paschall, 2007)

P-selectin is a 140 kDa glycoprotein expressed from platelet secreting granules and endothelial cell Weibel-Palade. Within several minutes, on histamin or thrombin stimulation, granules combine with plasma membranes, causing P-selectin to be expressed to the surface. Due to immediate induction and internalisation through endocytosis, P-selectin is estimated to mediate early levels of leukocyte rolling. In a matter of hours, P-selectin could also be regulated through transcription, resulting in chronic expression, a state of which plays a role in artherosclerosis (Paschall, 2007).

E-selectin, a 64 kDa glycoprotein, expresses endothelial cells (although not inconstitutively). E-selectin is regulated by cytokinee trancriptions, including tumor necrosis factor (TNF-α) and interleukin-1 (IL-1). Cytokine stimulation causes peak E-selectin expressions in 4 hours and recovering decrease in the subsequent 24 hours (Paschall, 2007).

L-selectin is a 75-110kDa molecular weighing glycoprotein (depending upon cell type), constitutively expressed in majority of leukocyte microvillous ends (except T memeory and natural killer (NK) cell groups). Molecular weight varaiability has been reported to be a result of L-selectin coding for 37 kDA core proteins with 8 possible sites for N-linked glycosylation. L-selectin is important in binding lymphocytes to high endothelial venules (HEV) and neutrophil invading inflammatory sites. On activating neutrophils, L-selectin is disrupted by proteolytic enzymes adjacent to transmembrane domains and released from the surface. High concentrations of released or dissolved L-selectin, may inhibit leukocyte attachment to the endothel. Cellular binded and dissolved forms of L-selectins have been associated with several diseases, including HIV, type 2 Diabetes, Kawasaki syndrome, leukemia, lymphoma, multiple sclerosis, neonatal bacterial infection, sepsis and stroke (Paschall, 2007).

Selectin Ligands

Selectin has a large amount of ligand candidates, however, only P-selectin glycoprotein ligand 1 (PSGL-1) has been extensivelly studied on molecular, cellular, and functional levels. A study using PSGL-1 coding gene-deficient knock outed rats showed delayed neutrophil recruitment resulting in moderate neutrophil counts (3 time increase), equivalent to P-selectin deficient rats. Apart from being responsibe for 90% of P-selectin binding, PSGL-1 is also the most essential ligand-1 during inflammatory states, from which PSGL-1 is presented by readily attached leukocytes and leukocyte fragments. Although not a main E-selectin ligand, PSGL-1 also binds to E-selectin. L-selectin ligands have been identified in secondary lymphatic high endothelial venules and are collectively recognized as peripheral node addressins (PNAd). From this group, podocalyxin is the most possible mediataing ligand for L-selectin to facilitate lymphocte entry to lymphatic nodes (Ley, 2003).

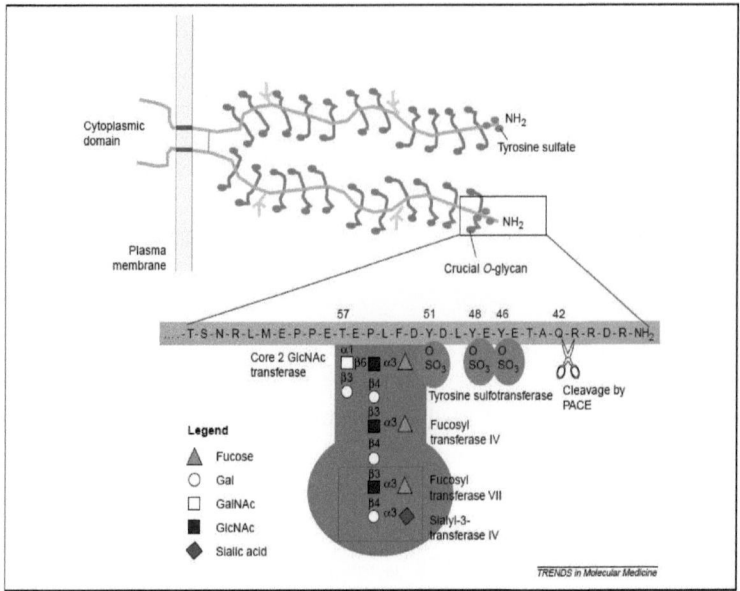

Figure 5. Homodimer structure of Human P-Selectin Glycoprotein Ligand 1 (PSGL-1). N-terminal tyrosine sulfates (violet) follwed by a tall glycoprotein spine much O-linked carbohydrates (dark green) and several N-linked carbohydrats (yellow). A functionally essential O-glycan (crutial) is shown. Stabilizing disulfid bindings (S-S) (vertical orange line) located near the plasma membran, and transmembran domain (red) and short cytoplasmic tail is also shown. Below, amino acid sequence of 38 residues are shown with tirosin sulfat (violet) and crucial O-glycans on T57 (dark green) and typical Carbohydrate side-chains are shown, with the associated type shown by Greek letters and responsible enzymes shown besides the next association. Sialyl Lewisx cluster (minimal selectin recognition) motives are highlighted in a red box. Mature PSGL-1 is brocken down by PACE, furin-like protease on Q42. Gal=galactosamin; GalNAc=N-asethylgalactosamine; GlcNAc=N-asetilglukosamine (Ley, 2003)

Inflamation/Leukocyte Recruitment

Leukocyte recruitment from intravascular compartments to inflammatory tissues protect the vertebrae from invading microorganisms and other external interferences. Leucoytes are recruited through a tightly regulated multi level adhesion cascade, consisting of the following phases (Sperandio et al., 2005; Oda et al, 1992):

1. Leukocyte capture

On identifying pathogens and pathogen activation, activated tissue macrophages release cytokinees, including IL-1, TNF-α dan kemokin. IL-1 dan

TNF-α causing vasular endothels adjacent to inflammatory sites to express cellular adhesion molecules, including Selectin. Circulating leukocytes are retrieved to inflammatory sites by chemokinees.

2. Rolling adhesion

   Circulating leukocyte carbohydrate ligands bind selectine molecules to inner sides of vasculatares with low affinity, causing slow movements of leukocytes. Subsequently, leukocytes role along the vascular wall, during which, transient binding is dormed and disrupted between selectins and ligands.

3. Tight adhesion

   At the same time, chemokinees are released by rolling leukocyte-activated macrophages and cause changes in surface integrins from a low affinity to a high affinity state. This is mediated by coinciding integrin activities by chemokinees and dissolved factors released by endothelial cells, causing leukocytes to bind to endothelial walls with high affinity. As a result, despite ongoing shear forces, leukocytes undergo immobilization.

4. Transmigration

   Leukocyte cytoskeletons are organized in such a manner that leukocytes are distributed though out the endothelial surface. In this form, leukocytes form psuedopodia and penetrate gaps between endothelial cells. Leucocyte transmigration occur due to PECAM proteins, found in leukocyte and endothelial cell superficies, effectively interacting and attracting leukocytes through the endothelium. Leukocytes secrete basal membrane degrading proteases, facilitating vascular expulsion, a process known as diapedesis. On entering interstitial spaces, leukocytes migrate along the chemotaxis radients towards inflammatory sites.

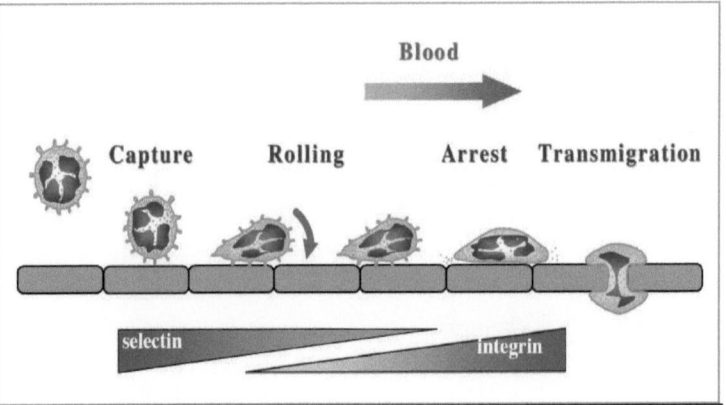

Figure 6. Leukocyte Adhesion Cascade. A leukocyte is captured from circulating system and then rolled along the vascular wall. Both processes are meditaed by selectins. Chemokinee signaling from surrounding tissues start transision from rolling to strong adhesions, halting, and then migrate. Strong adhesions are controlled by integrins (Paschall, 2007)

Role of Macrophages

Mononuclear phagocytes (monocytes and macrophages) are observed in most tissues and play a vital role in the innate and acquired immune system. Circulating monocytes produced by myeloid progenitor bone marrows are precursors for tissue macrophages. On release to the peripheral circulating system, monocytes circulate for several minutes to several days before entering tissues. Monocytes differentiate in to morphologically and functionally heterogenic effector cells, including retained macrophages left in inflammatory tissues and macrophages (Valentine, 2003)

Retained tissue macrophages perform certain necessary functions for each different anatomical site. Several example include: alveolar macrophages in the lungs, responsible for local defense against pathogens and particular materials; epidermal Langerhans cells; osteoclasts for bone remodelling; splenic macrophages and Kupffer cell located in the liver; supporting blood-originating pathogen clearance (Valentine, 2003).

During inflammatory responses, monocytes are recruited to injured tissues by attaching to vascular endothels and follow a local haptotactic and chemotactic gradient before differentiating in to macrophages. "Good" retained tissues or recent macrophages are main sources for chemokinees in injured tissues, and maybe instrumental in recruiting subsequent additional macrophages (Valentine, 2003).

Conventional knowledge has it that mononuclear macrophage follow neutrophils to inflammatory sites, phagocytize cellular debris and foreign bodies, and finally escape these sites. Prolonged presence of high mononuclear macrophage counts in recovering tissues usually indicate chronic inflamation by formation of granulated tissues that eventually result in necrosis, granuloma formation, fibrosis with encapsulation, and/or several degrees of scar tissue formation. Advanced studies reveal that macrophages indicate plasticity, defined as macrophage phenotype changes depending on local enviroment. Although classically (M1 macrophages) or alternatively (M2 macrophages) activated, substantial hetereogenicity exits between macrophage phenotyopes, due the wide functional scope it has on inflammatory responses and mantaining tissue homeostasis (Corna et al., 2010; Valentine, 2003). This paper would elucidate macrophage phenotype profiles in peritoneal tissues of endometriosis patients as means of obtaining a more accurate and complete description of host immunity responses.

Macrophage is a key element in non-specific immunity response, as part of the antigen non-specific immunity system that does not involve immunologic memory. Macrophages defend host through recognizing, phagocytizing, and destructing invading microorgansims and also funtions as scavengers, aiding to clear apoptotic cells and cellular debris. Macrophages secrete various self-facilitating functioning cytokines, growth factors, enzymes, and prostaglandins, while simultaneously stimulating other cell type growth and proliferation. Macrophages normally reside in peritoneal fluid and undergo increased activities in endometriosis women. Rather than acting as scavengers (M1 macrophages) to eliminate ectopic endometrial cells, alternatively activated peritoneal macrophages (M2 macrophages) and circulating monocytes in women with endometriosis seem to support endometriosis by secreting growth factors and cytokines that stimulate ectopic endometrial proliferation and inhibit scavenging functions (Fritz et al., 2011).

Studies on expmerimental rats showed that alternatively activated macrophages (M2 macrophages) dramatically increase growth of endometriosis lesions in rat. Whereas inflammatory macrophages (M1 macroohages) effectively protect rats from endometriosis. Therefore, endogen macrophages involved in tissue remodelling seem to play a role in the natural course of endometriosis necessary to form effective vascularisation and growth of endometriosis lesions (Allavena et al., 2008; Bacci et al., 2009).

Alternatively activating macrophages (M2 macrophages) is a key step in the development of endometriosis, in which increased M2 macrophages would secrete and enhance cytokines, prostaglandins, components, and growth factors (tumor necrosis factor-β (TNF-α), IL-6, and transforming growth factor-β (TGF-β)) concentrations. Normally, endometriosis cells entering the peritoneal cavity are eliminated by macrophages. Aberrations in endometriosis results in an ineffective immunological clearing system to foreign bodies. Apart from neovascularization, M2 macrophages and increased levels of cytokinees also result in endometrial cellular initiation, progression, and growth (Gupta et al, 2006).

Consequently, M2 macrophages are more significantly involved in the pathogenesis of endometriosis. This maybe caused by genetic, hormonal, and enviromental factors. A study showed that estrogen increases M2 macrophage activities through surface expressing estrogen receptors. Under estrogen effects, M2 macrophages secrete cytokines and growth factors (VEGF, hepatocyte growth factors, and TNF-α), thus contributing to the development and persistance of endometriosis (Montagna et al, 2008).

Macrophage phenotypes could be characterized as proinflammatory macrophages (M1 macroophages) or immunomodulatory macrophages or tissue remodelling macrophages (M2 macroophages). Immunohistological methods could be employed to identify macrophage surface markers, consisting of CD68, CD80 and CCR7 (M1 profile), and CD163 (M2 profile). (Badylak et al, 2008).

Genetic Factors

In humans and non-human primates, endometriosis tend to group in families. This disease is frequently observed in monozygotic and dizygotic twins and has similar age onsets in non twin female siblings. Endometriosis has a 6 to 7 higher occurence rate in first level family members of patients than general population. These observations indicate that endometriosis is genetically based and predisposition factors are inherited as complex genetic charecteristics, the phenotypes of which reflect inter allele variations of susceptible genes and enviromental factors. A world collaborative project (the Oxford Endometriosis Gene Study) involving DNA systematic analysis of biological families and parents of patients with endometriosis has been organized to identify genes that possibly affect the events of endometriosis (Fritz et al., 2011).

Possible predisposing genes for endometriosis comprises genes involved in molecular processes that control survival of released endometrial cells, peritoneal cellular attachment and invasion, proliferation, neovascularization, or inflammatory response. Eutopic endometrium in endometriosis subjects are also resistent to apoptosis and may also show abnormal cell adhesion molecule expressions (Fritz et al., 2011).

Complex Diseases: Genetics

Diseases not compliant to the Classical Mendelian inheriting system are known as Complex diseases. They are relatively frequent in general population and seem to to group in families. In addition, complex diseases are known to be affected by several genetic and enviromental factors, as well as the interaction between the two. General variant hypothesis states that common genetic variants with relatively high frequencies, but with low penetrance, is the main contributor to this disease (Altshuler et al., 2008). However, a rare variant, with low frequencies and high frequencies has also reported similar contributions. Genetic etiology is most frequently based on the combination of rare and common variants (Stratton and Rahman, 2008; Sundqvist, 2011).

Gene Polymorphsme in Genomes

Genetic polymorphisme is the difference of DNA sequences between individuals, groups, or population. The main source for these discrepancies are SNPs, *sequence repeats*, insetion, deletion and recombination (Kaleigh, 2002). SNPs are the source for genome variety and are mutations from a single base. SNPs are the most simple and common form of genetic polymorphism in the human genome (90% of all human polymorphism) (Kaleigh, 2002).

Although known to have 99,9% identical genome DNA, a substantial amount of variations have been observed in the human genome. Genetic variations may explain various phenotypes between individuals, although most variants are believed to be neutral with no phenotypic effect. SNPs are the most common genetic variation, in which nucleotides are replaced, inserted, or deleted. SNPs count in human genome is estimated at 3.3 million with an average of 1 SNP in 1000 bases. SNPs are located in coding and non-coding regions (Altshuler et al., 2008; Frazer et al., 2009). Synonymous SNPs, located in coding regions, may cause amino acid alterations, frame shifts, or translational termination, therefore effecting functions at the protein level. SNPs may also have no effect on amino acid sequences. As they are located in regulator elements (gene promoters, enhancers, and silencers), SNPs located on the non-coding regions, known as non-synonymous SNPs, may also have functional effects (Daly et al., 2001; Sundqvist, 2011).

Genetic Polymorphism in Endometriosis

Several gene polymorphisms have been recognized to be involved in endometriosis, including inflammatory genes, steroid synthesis, hormonal receptors, growth factors, adhesion molecules, cellular cycle regulation, apoptosis, and oncogenesis. Interassociation between these inflammatory genes including IL-10, IL-2, IL-12, IL-16, IL-18, TGF-β, IFN-γ, TNF-α and TNF-β, have also beem observed. A study on Caucasion women reported that polymorphism was associated with the adhesion molecule, intercelluler adhesion molecule-I (ICAM I) (Tempfer et al., 2009).

Tables 2 to 5 all polymorphisms associated with endometriosis.

Table 2 Inflammatory Mediating Gen Polimorphism in Endometriosis (Tempfer et al., 2009)

Gene (Locus, Protein Name And Its Function)	Variant Name	dbSNP ID
CCL5 [17q11.2-q12, chemokinee (C–C motif) ligand 5 (RANTES): chemokinee]	-403G/A	rs2107538
	-28C/G	rs2280788
CCR2 (3p21.31, monocyte chemotactic protein 1 receptor: chemokinee receptor)	p.V64I	rs1799864
CCR5 (3p21.31, chemokinee (C–C motif) receptor 5: chemokinee receptor)	Delta32 (32 bp deletion)	rs333
CDH1 (16q22.1, epithelial cadherin 1: adhesion molecule)	PmlI RFLP (3'- UTR C/T)	rs1801026

24

	-160C/A	rs1620
	-347G/GA	rs5030625
CDKN1A (6p21.2, cyclin-dependent kinase inhibitor 1A (p21): regulation of cell cycle)	p.S31R	rs1801270
CTLA4 (2q33, cytotoxic T lymphocyte antigen-4: T-cell ligand)	49A/G	rs231775
	CT60A/G	rs3087243
EGFR (7p12, epidermal growth factor receptor: regulates cell growth and differentiation)	2073A/T	rs17337023
FAS (10q24.1, FAS: mediates apoptosis)	-1377G/A	rs2234767
	-670A/G	rs1800682
FASLG (1q23, FAS ligand: mediates apoptosis)	-844C/T	rs763110
HLA-A (6p21.3, human leukocyte antigen-A: major histocompatibility I protein)	HLA-A	
HLA-B (6p21.3, human leukocyte antigen-B: major histocompatibility I protein)	HLA-B	
HLA-DPB1 (6p21.3, human leukocyte antigen DP b1: major histocompatibility II protein)	HLA-DPB1*01-*03, *0401-*0402, *05, *06, *08-*11, *13-*19	
HLA-DQB1 (6p21.3, human leukocyte antigen DQ b1: major histocompatibility II protein)	HLA-DQB1*0201, *0301-*0303, *0401-*0402, *0501-*0503, *0601-*0604	

HLA-DRB1 (6p21.3, human leukocyte antigen DR b1: major histocompatibility II protein)	HLA-DRB1*0101, *0301, *0401-*0408, *0410, *0701, *0801-*0803, *09, *10, *1101, *1104, *1201-*1202, *1301-*1302, *1401, *1402, *1404, *1405, *1501, *1502, *1602 (+*0102, *0103, *0302, *0804, *1602, *1305 in Japanese study) (+*1111, *1339, *1406, *1407, *1412 in Korean study)	
ICAM1 (19p13.3-p13.2, intercellular adhesion molecule-1: adhesion molecule)	p.G241R	rs1799968
	p.K469E	rs5498
IFNG (12q14, interferon-g: cytokinee)	CA repeat	
IGF2 (11p15.5, insulin-likegrowth factor II: cytokinee)	ApaI RFLP (17 200G/A)	rs680
IL4 (5q31.1, interleukin-4: cytokinee)	-590C/T	rs2243250
	70 bp VNTR	

	(intron 3)	
IL6 (7p21, interleukin-6: cytokinee)	-174G/C	rs1800795
	-634C/G (-572C/G)	rs1800796
IL10 (1q31-q32, interleukin-10: cytokinee)	-1082G/A	rs1800896
	-627A/C (-592C/A)	rs1800872
IL18 (11q22.2-q22.3, interleukin-18: cytokinee)	105A/C	rs549908
IL1B (2q14, interleukin-1b: cytokinee)	-511C/T	rs16 944
	3953C/T	rs1143634
IL1R1 (2q11.2, interleukin-1 receptor 1: cytokinee receptor)	PstI RFLP	rs2041748
	BsrBI RFLP	No dbSNP ID
IL2RB (22q13.1, interleukin-2 receptor b: cytokinee receptor)	881T/C	rs228953
IL1RN (2q14.2, interleukin-1R antagonist: cytokinee)	86 bp VNTR (intron 2)	
IL12RB1 (19p13.1, interleukin-12 receptor b: cytokinee receptor)	p.G378R	rs401502
NOS3 (7q36, endothelial nitric oxide synthase: catalyses synthesis of nitric oxide, a pro-inflammatory molecule)	p.E298D	rs1799983
TGFB1 (19q13.1, transforming growth factor b1: cytokinee)	-509C/T	rs1800469
TNF (6p21.3, tumour necrosis factor a: cytokinee)	-1031T/C	rs1799964
	-863C/A	rs1800630
	-857C/T	rs1799724
	-308G/A	rs1800629
	-238G/A	rs361525

		rs1800750,
		rs3093661,
		rs1800610,
		rs3093662,
		rs4645843,
		rs3093664,
		rs3091257
TNF (6p21.3, tumour necrosis factor β (Lymphotoxin-alpha LTA): cytokinee)	Intron 1+252A/G (A1069G)	rs909253
		rs2857602,
		rs2844486,
		rs3131637,
		rs2844484,
		rs2844483,
		rs4647191,
		rs2844482,
		rs2071590,
		rs1800683,
		rs2239704,
		rs909253,
		rs2857713,
		rs3093543,
		rs1041981
TNFRSF1B (1p36.3-p36.2, tumour necrosis factor receptor 2: cytokinee receptor)	p.M196R	rs1061622
TP53 (17p13.1, tumour protein p53: regulation of cell cycle)	p.R72P	rs1042522

Table 3 Sex Hormone and Hormone Regulator Gene Polymorphism in Endometriosis (Tempfer et al., 2009)

Gene (Locus, Protein Name And Its Function)	Variant Name	dbSNP ID
AR (Xq11.2-q12, androgen receptor gene: hormone receptor)	CAG repeat (exon 1)	
ESR1 (6q25.1, estrogen receptor α: hormone receptor)	TA repeat (promoter)	
	PvuII RFLP (-397T/C) (IVS1 -401T/C)	rs2234693
	XbaI RFLP (-351A/G)	rs7340799
ESR2 (14q23.2, estrogen receptor β: hormone receptor)	RsaI RFLP (1082G/A)	rs1256049
	AluI RFLP (1730A/G)	rs4986938
NRIP1 (21q11.2, receptor interacting protein 140: estrogen and progesterone receptor cofactor)	p.R448G	rs2229742
PGR (11q22-q23, progesterone receptor: hormone receptor)	331A/G	rs10895068
	PROGINS (320 bp PV/HS-1 Alu insertion in intron G and 2 SNPs: rs1042838 in exon 4 and rs104839 in exon 5)	

Table 4 Metabolism and Biosynthesis Enzyme Gene Polymorphysm in Endometriosis (Tempfer et al., 2009)

Gene (Locus, Protein Name And Its Function)	Variant	
	Name	dbSNP ID
AHR (7p15, arylhydrocarbon receptor: transcription factor, detoxification)	p.K554R	rs2066853
ARNT (7p15, arylhydrocarbon receptor nuclear translocator: transcription factor, detoxification)	567G/C (p.V189V)	rs2228099
AHRR (5p15.3, arylhydrocarbon receptor repressor: transcription factor repressor, detoxification)	p.A185P	rs2292596
COMT (22q11.21, catechol-O-methyl transferase: steroid biosynthesis, Estrogen metabolism)	p.V158M	rs4680
CYP1A1 (15q22-q24, cytochrome P450 1A1 enzyme: steroid biosynthesis, Estrogen metabolism, phase I detoxification)	MspI RFLP (6235T/ C) (3801T/C) (m1)	rs4646903
	p.I462V 4889A/G (m2)	rs1048943
CYP1B1 (2p21, cytochrome P450 1B1 enzyme: steroid biosynthesis, Estrogen metabolism, phase I detoxification)	p.N453S	rs1800440
	p.L432V, p.D449D(C/T), p.N453S, p.A119S	rs1056836, rs1056837, rs1800440, rs1056827
CYP17A1 (10q24.3, cytochrome	MspA1 RFLP	rs743572

P450 17 enzyme: estrogen biosynthesis)	(234T/C)	
CYP19A1 (15q21.1, aromatase: steroid biosynthesis)	TTTA repeat microsatellite	
	p.R264C	rs28757190
GSTM1 (1p13.3, glutathione-S-transferase M1: phase II detoxification)	Null deletion	
GSTP1 (11q13, glutathione-S-transferase P1: phase II detoxification)	p.I105V	rs1695
GSTT1 (22q11.23, glutathione-S-transferase T1: phase II detoxification)	Null deletion	
HSD17B1 (17q11-q21, 5 17-b hydroxysteroid dehydrogenase: testosterone biosynthesis, Estrogen metabolism)	-27A/C (vIV)	
	p.S312G	rs605059
MPO (17q23.1, myeloperoxidase: phase I detoxification, oxidation and activation of carcinogens and nitric oxide)	-463G/A	rs2333227
NAT1 (8p23.1-p21.3, N-acetyltransferase 1: phase II detoxification)	NAT1*3, *4, *10, *11	
NAT2 (8p22, N-acetyltransferase 2: phase II detoxification)	Nat2*4-*7	

Table 5 Glucose Homeostasis Gene Polimorphism, Vascular functions, Tissue Remodelling in Endometriosis (Tempfer et al., 2009)

Gene (Locus, Protein Name And Its Function)	Variant	
	Name	dbSNP ID
Mediators of glucose homeostasis		
GALT (9p13, galactose-1-phosphate uridyl transferase: galactose metabolism)	p.N314D	rs2070074
	p.Q188R	No dbSNP ID (rare mutation
PPARG (3p25, peroxisome proliferator-activated receptor-g: transcription factor; mediates insulin resistance, regulates CCL5 expression)	p.P12A	rs1801282
	p.H447H, 161C/T	rs3856806
Mediators of vascular function or genes linked to cardiovascular risk		
ACE (17q23.3, angiotensin-I converting enzyme: mediates vascular homeostasis)	-240A/T	rs4291
	2350A/G	rs4343
	287 bp ALU ins/del in intron 16	Several dbSNP IDs: rs4646994 or rs4340, rs1799752
COL18A1 (21q22.3, endostatin: inhibits endothelial cell proliferation and angiogenesis)	4349G/A (p.D1437 N) (p.D104 N)	rs12483377
VEGFA (6p12, vascular endothelial	405G/C	Rs2010963

growth factor: mediates vascular permeability and angiogenesis)	(-634G/C)	
	-460C/T	Rs833061
	936C/T	rs3025039
Genes involved in tissue remodelling		
AHSG (3q27, alpha 2-Heremans Schmidt glycoprotein: mediates tissue development)	p.T230M	rs4917
	p.T238S	rs4918
MMP1 (11q22.3, matrix metalloproteinase-1: tissue remodelling)	-1607ins/ delG (1G/2G)	rs112925
MMP3 (11q22.3, matrix metalloproteinase-3: tissue remodelling)	-1171ins/ delA (5A/6A)	
MMP7 (11q21-q22, matrix metalloproteinase-7: tissue remodelling)	-181A/G	rs1799750
MMP9 (20q11.2-q13.1, matrix metalloproteinase-9: tissue remodelling)	-1562C/T	rs3918242
SERPINE1 (7q21.3–q22, plasminogen activator inhibitor-1: fibrinolysis system. Linked to cardiovascular disease)	2675ins/delG (4G/5G)	Several dbSNP IDs: rs1799768, rs34857375, rs1799762, rs1799889
Genes involved in signal transduction		
EMX2 (10q26.1, empty spiracles homeobox 2: homeodomain transcription factor)		rs1860399, rs82 613, rs82 612, rs242956,

		rs703409, rs703411, rs1638626, rs2286629, rs385209, rs855769, rs365446, rs8192640, rs740734, rs855768, rs2240776, rs703413, rs4751627, rs242960, rs8181280, rs855766, rs4752078, rs4752079
STAT6 (12q13, signal transducer and activator of transcription 6: signal transduction and activation of transcription)	2964G/A	rs324015
Genes involved in malignant transformation		
KRAS (12p12.1, kirsten rat sarcoma viral oncogene homologue: proto-oncogene)		rs7304896, rs7132980, rs4556643, rs11612828, rs12320328, rs11047921, rs11047919, rs7309670, rs17388893,

	rs10842514,
	rs6487464,
	rs4495968,
	rs17388587,
	rs11047912,
	rs17329025,
	rs17388148,
	rs11047901,
	rs12579073,
	rs12313763,
	rs1137282,
	rs9266,
	rs13096,
	rs11047892,
	rs4963857,
	rs7137734,
	rs11047889,
	rs11047887,
	rs11609324,
	rs11836162,
	rs3924649
PTEN (10q23.3, phosphate and	rs2673836,
tensin	rs1234220,
homologue: tumour suppressor)	rs1234219,
	rs1903858,
	rs2299939,
	rs11202597,
	rs1234224,
	rs2735343,
	rs17431184,
	rs555895,
	rs2736627,
	rs926091,
	rs532678,

| | rs701848, |
| | rs478839 |

A study comparing L-selectin gen profile expressions in rat endometriosis tissues and healthy eutopic human endometrium, analysed using cDNA microarray, quantitative real time RT-PCR, showed that endometriosis tissues have a 46 time higher L-selectin trancript level than healthy eutopic rat endometrium. This study concluded that L-selectin played a significant role in the pathogenesis of endometriosis. Seventy five and 45 gene expressions were upregulated and downregulated, respectively, than eutopic endometrial tissues. Several genes were more distinctly expressed than others. Gene transcriptions for osteopontine, Lyn, Vav1, Runx1, and L-selectin in endometriosis lesions were 130, 10, 10, 12 and 46 higher than the eutopic endometrium (Konno et al., 2007). Gene Polymorphism may also occur in L-selectin in association with the occurence of endometriosis.

Several types of L-selectin polymorphism have been reported in association with other auto immune disease, including L-selectin gene polymorphism (a C/T transision in exon 6) in spinal muscular atrophy (Stavarachi et al., 2009), L-selectin gen F206L polymorphism in Celiac disease (Kaur et al., 2006) and ischemic stroke (Wei et al., 2011).

Table 6

	Disease association	Polymorphism
Hajilooi M., et al. 2006	Coronary Artery Disease	F206L
Kaur G., et al. 2006	Celiac Disease	F206L
Liu J., et al. 2012	Diabetes Mellitus Tipe-2 dan Insulin Resistensi	P213S
Stavarachi et al. 2009	Spinal Muscular atrophy	P213S
Wei Y, et al, 2011	Stroke Iskemik	P213S
Rafei A., et. al. 2006	Brucellosis	F206L
Khazen D., et al. 2009	Inflammatory Bowel Disease	F206L

| Russell A., et al., 2005 | Systemic Lupus Erythematosus | F206L |
| Chen HY., et al. 2007 | Graves' Disease | P213S |

L-selectin gen is located in chromosome 1 locus q23-q25, and consists of 28.038 pairs of nucleotide base arranged by 10 exons (Iida et al., 2003).

Chapter 3
Methodology

This comparative analytical, two population case-control study was approved by the health research ethical committee of North Sumatera c/o Medical School, University of Sumatera Utara and was conducted at the Department of Obstetrics and Gynecolocy at Haji Adam Malik General Hospital, Dr. Pirngadi Medan Hospital, networking hospitals and private clinics throughout Medan from January 2013 - March 2014 until the minimum required amount of samples was obtained. Reproductive aged women, complaining menstrual pain, abdominal located bulging, and/or infertility, visiting the Gynecology outpatient clinics at Haji Adam Malik General Hospital, Dr. Pirngadi Medan Hospital, networking hospitals and private hospitals throughout Medan, comprised the study population, from which patients suspected with endometriosis based on a history taking, physical and sonographic examination and meeting inclusion criterias were taken as samples through consecutive sampling. Sample size was statistically determined ($\alpha = 0,05$ → $Z_\alpha=1,96$ dan $\beta = 0,20$ → $Z_\beta=0,84$), from which the case and control group were both allocated with 22 samples each. The case group comprised of women diagnosed with endometriosis whereas the control group consisted of non endometriosis women.

This study aimed on determining an association betweeen L–selectin gene P213S polymorphism with cases of endometriosis, using M1 and M2 macrophage profiles/ratios as intermediating variables between the two. Previous studies showed that potentially disrupting factors include history of ischemic stroke, spinal muscular atrophy, and celiac disease and were consequently considered exclusion criterias.

Two hypotheseses were proposed. The first, L–selectin gene P213S polymorphism was hypothesized to be associated with the events of endometriosis, whereas the second was to propose a role discrepancy between M1 and M2 macrophages in the pathogenesis of endometriosis.

Twenty to 45 year old women, laparascopicsally/laparatomically and histopataholologically confirmed diagnosed with endometriosis, with irregular menstrual cycles and also willing to participate after filling a written informed consent form, were included in the case group. Twenty to 45 year old women, laparascopicsally/laparatomically and histopataholologically confirmed not diagnosed with endometriosis, eg., cases of self requested tubectomy, regular menstrual cycles, and also willing to participate after filling a written informed consent form were assigned to the control group.

Gynecological disorders, including non endometriosis ovarian cyst, ovarian tumor, and uterine myomas, endocrine disorders, currently on hormonal medication for minimally 3 months prior to recruitment, with a previous pelvic surgery, history ischemic stroke, muscular spinal atrophy, and Celiac disease, or patients who self withdrew, were excluded from the study.

Visiting patients at the gynecology outpatient clinic were taken a complete history, and then underwent physical/gynecological and sonographic examinations to determine an indication (including history of infertility, dysmenorrhea, self requested tubectomy, endometriosis cyst, etc) to perform a laparoscopy/laparotomy, and if present, a laparoscopy was scheduled to take place during the menstrual cycle of the proliferation phase.

The presence of endometriosis was assessed during laparoscopy/laparotomy and was further confirmed by histopathologically examining peritoneal tissues. Laparoscopy is an endoscopic procedure that directly visualizes the peritoneal cavity using a small telescope. Endometriosis was defined as extra uterine ectopic endometrial glands or stromas, the presence of which were confirmed laparascopically or histopathologically. Patients diagnosed with endometriosis were included in the case group, after which severity was assessed based on the Revised Classification of Endometriosis, American Society For Reproductive Medicine (ASRM), 1997 (see fig. 1), which is as follows : stage I (minimal degree) : ASRM score 1-5, stage II (mild degree) : ASRM score 6-15, stage III (moderate degree) : ASRM score 16-40, and stage IV (severe degree) : ASRM score >40.

Non endometriosis patients were categorized in to the control group based on inclusion and exclusion criterias. During the procedure (laparoscopy/laparotomy), peritoneal tissues were sampled and 5 cc blood taken by venous punctures from the ante cubiti vein area. DNA isolation and genotyping was performed on these samples, whereas peritoneal tissue samples were histopathologically and immunohistochemically examined by semi-quantitative percentage of cells (Score 0: 0%; 1: 1-25%; 2: 26-50%; 3: 51-75%; 4: >75%).

Histopathological and Imunohistochemical Examination of Peritoneal Tissues

Peritoneal tissue samples were examined at the Pathology Laboratory, Medical Faculty, University of Sumatera. During the procedure, peritoneal tissues of endometriosis and non endometriosis samples were biopsied and fixated using 10% buffer formalin. Fixated tissues were dehydrated by alcohol for 1 hour and 30 minutes, and then cleared using xylene, from which paraffin block were made. These blocks were then cut into 4 μm thick pieces, inserted into a water bath, and subsequently placed on a previously glycerine spreaded object glass. Specimens were then defarafinized using xylol, rehydrated with alcohol, rinsed with streaming water, and stained using Haemotoxyline-Eosine. These specimens were histopatahologically examined under a light microscope with a 400 time magnification, immunohistochemically proccessed using monoclonal mouse anti-human-CD68 (Clone PG-M1) and anti-CD163 (Dako) (BD Pharmingen) staining, and then rinsed using Tris Buffered saline (TBS) pH 7,4. DAB was then combined with a chromogene solution and was diluted with the following ratio : 20 μL DAB : 1000 μL substrate. On cleaning with streaming water, specimens were counterstained using haematoxylin and 5% lithium carbonate, and cleaned again with streaming water, after which samples were dehydrated with alcohol and cleared with xylol. Samples were then microscopically examined. Immunoprecipitated areas of M1 and M2 macrophage cells [with anti-human-CD68 mouse monoclonal markers (Clone PG-M1) and anti-CD163 presented peritoneal tissue slices] were calculated in antigen percentages.

Macrophage (M0) was defined as a monocyte originated macrophage. Main types include: peritoneal and alveolar macrophages; hystiocytes; liver Kupffer cells, and osteoclasts. These macrophages function in non specific (innate) and specific (cell-mediated) immunity systems and by fagositizing cellular and pathogen debris, acting as both stationary or mobile cells, and also stimulating lymphocytes and other immune cells to respond against pathogens. M1 macrophage is a macrophage induced by the classical profile activation triggered by microbial products, including LPS or TH1 cytokinees (IFN--γ and TNF-α). M1 macrophage synthesizes and releases pro-inflammatory factors, including IL-1β, IL-6, IL-12, and TNF-α, producing high concentrated NO and reactive oxygen intermediates (ROIs), and type-1 chemochins, such as CXCL-10, CXCL-11, and CCL5. M1 macrophages are associated with microbial activities, tumor resistance, and cytotoxic tissue damage.

Under stimulation by specific cytokines, eg. IL-4, IL-10, IL-13, and non GM-CSF M-CSF, LPS, INF, etc, M2 macrophages alter the inflammatory and adaptive immune proccess, thus promoting cell proliferation by producing growth factors and arginase pathway products, engulf debris by expressing scavenger receptors, and support angiogenesis, tissue remodelling and regeneration, suppress the adaptive immunity system and support endomteriosis growth. CD-163 is a Hemoglobin/haptoglobin complex scavenger receptor, expressed dominantly by M2 macrophages. CD-68 (Clone PG-M1): M1 macrophage surface marker.

DNA Isolation

During laparoscopy, 500 µL peripheral blood samples were taken from case and control groups by venous punctures from the antecubiti vein, from which DNA was extracted and analyzed. Genom DNA was extracted using a High Pure PCR Templete Preparation Kit (Roche Applied Biosystem) and then restored using an EDTA anticoagulant at 4°C, until used for analysis.

DNA is a polimere of deoxyrybonucletide units. A nucleotide consists of a nitrogen base, one glucose and one more phosphate sequence. The genome is defined as the most comprehensive complement of human DNA.

Genotyping

L-selectin gene P213S polymorphism genotyping was examined using the PCR-RFLP method. PCR is a technique used to amplify small fragments or DNA areas into sufficiently larger particles adequate for analysis, using electrophoresis and blotting. These fragments were amplified in a Perkin Elmer Gene Amp PCR system 2400, in 25 µL reaction volumes containing 200 ng genome DNA, 200 µM for every dATP, dCTP, dGTP, dTTP, 50 mM KCl, 10 mM Tris-HCl, 3mM $MgCl_2$, 0,5 µM from each primary, and 1 unit Taq polimerase (FastStart Taq DNA Polymerase, dNTPPack, Roche Applied Biosystem). The primary sequence was as follows: forward 5'-TGATTCAGTGTGAGCCTTTG-3' and reverse 5'-CTTGACAGGTTGGTTCTG-3'. The PCR reaction was performed in the following condition: 2 minutes at 94°C, 30 cycles for 1 minute at 94°C, 50 seconds at 59°C, 40 seconds at 72°C and 1 minute at 72°C.

Gen polymorphism was defined as inter various gene DNA sequences between individuals, groups, or populations. L-selectin gene P213S polymorphism gene is an

L-selectin gene polymorphism, in which the cytokine base is converted into thymin on codon number 213, causing the conversion of proline (P) into Serine (S).

PCR products (length 186 base pairs) were verified using agarosa gel electrophoresis (2%) and then digested for 3 hours using a 5 5 U/reaction Hph I enzyme (New England Biolabs, Inc. Beverly, USA), according to manufacturer instructions. On ethidium bromida staining, restricted products were visualized on the 8% polyacrilamide gel under ultraviolet light. DNA was isolated and genotyped at the Medan Prodia Laboratory in cooperation with the Eijkman Molecular Biology Institute, Jakarta.

Data were univariately and bivariately analyzed. Descriptive data were univariately analyzed. Using bivariate analysis, variables were analyzed using a chi-square test (a p value<0,05 was considered statistically significant) to compare genotype distribution of polymorphism and macrophage profiles between case and control groups.

Chapter 4
Results

On histopathologically confirming endometriosis in patients who previously underwent laparotomy/laparoscopy at Haji Adam Malik General Hospital, Permata Bunda Hospital, and Stella Maris Hospital from Januray 2013-March 2014, 23 subjects were enrolled and assigned to the case group. Whereas, 23 non endometriosis subjects, previously undergoing a laparoscopic tubectomy at the Mantap Sterilisation Clinic, Medan and confirmed with no peritoneal or reproductive organ lesions of endometriosis, were assigned to the control group. Blood samples were taken preoperatively and only non endometriosis tissues were histopataologically and immunohistochemically examined.

Subjects Demographic Characteristics

Demographic characteristics are shown in table 1. Endometriosis and non endometriosis subjects were averagely aged 32,83 and 35,48 years old, respectively. The case group was dominated by stage 4 endometriosis patients (69,9%). No cases of stage endometriosis were encountered. Ethnicity was diversed as subjects came from various areas.

Table 7 Subject Demographic Charecteristics

Charecteristics	Endometriosis	Non Endometriosis
Age, Mean (±SD)	32,83 (±6,827)	35,48 (±5,877)
Ethnic, n (%)		
Acehnese	2 (8,7)	2 (8,7)
Bataknese	9 (39,1)	5 (21,7)
Javanese	8 (34,8)	11 (47,8)
Indian	1 (4,3)	-
Malay	1 (4,3)	2 (8,7)
Nias	1 (4,3)	1 (4,3)
Tionghoa	1 (4,3)	-
Minang	-	2 (8,7)
Endometriosis Stage, n (%)		
Stage 1	-	-

Stage 2	2 (8,7)	-
Stage 3	5 (21,7)	-
Stage 4	16 (69,6)	-

Distribution and Association between Genotype and P213S L-selectin allele

Table 8 displays genotype frequency rates of L-selectin gene P213S polymorphism in endometriosis and non-endometriosis subjects. 30,4%, 56,5%, and 13% endometriosis subjects had a PP, PS, and SS genotype, respectively whereas 60,9%, 39,1%, and 0% non-endometriosis subjects had a PP, PS, and SS L-selectin gene P213S polymorphism genotype, respectively. Chi-square tests showed that genotyping significantly differed between endometriosis and non endometriosis subjects, with a p value of 0,048.

Tabel 8 Association between genotype and cases of endometriosis

Genotypes	Subjects		p*
	Endometriosis	Non Endometriosis	
PP	7 (30,4%)	14 (60,9%)	0,048
PS	13 (56,5%)	9 (39,1%)	
SS	3 (13%)	0 (0%)	
Total	23 (100%)	23 (100%)	

*Chi-square test

This study focused on the P and S allele (of L-selectin gene P213S polymorphismgene) and the possible associated role in developing endometriosis, assuming that the P coversion to S would increase incidence rates of this disease. Results from table 9 show that the S allele has higher frequency rates in endometriosis subjects than non endometriosis subjects (41,3% vs 19,6%). The P and S allele were correlated with the diagnosis of endometriosis, with correlation coefficients of 0,363 (pvalue 0,48) and 0,383 (p value 0,034), respectively.

Table 9 Association between L-selectin P213S allele and endometriosis

| Allele | Subjects | | R | p* |
	Endometriosis	Non Endometriosis		
P	27 (58,7%)	37 (80,4%)	0,363	0,048
S	19 (41,3%)	9 (19,6%)	0,383	0,034
Total	46 (100%)	46 (100%)		

Chi-square test

Assuming that the S allele is associated with increased rates of endometriosis, table 10 shows that S containing genotypes (PS and SS genotype) are more frequently encountered in the case groups than the control group (69,6% vs 39,1%). This fact also applies for endometriosis subjects, with higher incidence rates of S containing genotypes (PS and SS, 69,6%), than the P containing type (30,4%). Increased S allele containing genotype rates (PS and SS) in cases of L-selectin P213S gene polymorphism were significantly associated with events of endometriosis (p = 0,038).

Table 10 Association between PP and PS+SS L-selectin gene P213S polymorphism genotypes and endometriosis

| Genotypes | Subjects | | p* |
	Endometriosis	Non Endometriosis	
PP	7 (30,4%)	14 (60,9%)	0,038
PS + SS	16 (69,6%)	9 (39,1%)	
Total	23 (100%)	23 (100%)	

Chi-square test

Table 11 displays the extent of association between S alleles and events of endometriosis, from which the presence of this allele is associated with a 3 times higher risk of developing endometriosis (OR 2,893; IK 95% 1,135 - 7,373, p value 0,026). The results of this table also show that S allele carrier containing genotypes (SS and PS) have a 4 times higher risk than the PP genotype (OR 3,556; CI 95% 1,049 - 12,052, p value 0,04). Table 6 shows that PP, PS, and SS containing genotypes were dominantly staged 4 (37,5%, 43,8%, and 18,8% respectively), whereas all SS genotyped subjects had stage 4. Only 5 PS genotyped subjects had stage 3, whereas one PP and PS genotyped subject each were staged 2. On classifying endometriosis into two groups, minimal-mild and moderate-severe, no significant association was apparently established between severity degrees and P213S L-selectin gene genotypes, the results of which are displayed in table 13 (p value 1,0).

Table 11 Association between S allele and L-selectin gentype with cases of endometriosis

Subjects	p*	OR*	CI 95%
S Allele	0,026	2,893	1,135 – 7,373
PS + SS Genotype	0,041	3,556	1,049 – 12,052

Mantel-Haenszel Common Odds Ratio Estimate

Table 12 Distribution of endometriosis stages based on L-selectin P213S genotypes

Subjects	Genotype		
	PP	PS	SS
Stage 2	1 (50%)	1 (50%)	0 (0%)
Stage 3	0 (0%)	5 (100%)	0 (0%)
Stage 4	6 (37,5%)	7 (43,8%)	3 (18,8%)

Kolmogorov-Smirnov Z test

Table 13 Association between severity degrees of endometriosis and L-selectin P213s genotypes

Severity degrees of Endometriosis	Genotype			p*
	PP	PS	SS	
Minimal – Mild	1 (50%)	1 (50%)	0 (0%)	1,0
Moderate – Severe	6(28,6%)	12 (51,7%)	3 (14,3%)	

Distribution and Association between Macrophages and Endometriosis

Specimens were blindly immunohistochemically examined by two pathologists, from whom the clinical features of each group were with held. Table 14 shows kappa values of 92,6% and 100% for CD68 and CD163, respectively, indicating a high inter observer uniformity in assessing CD68 and CD 163 expression.

Table 14 Kappa value to Observer 1 and Observer 2

Observer Compatibility	Value	p value
CD68	0,926	0,0001
CD163	1,000	0,0001

Semi-quantitative immunohistochemical scoring shows that 21,72%, 26,1%, and 21,7% endometriosis subjects express CD68 +1, +2, and +3 macrophages, respectively (overall 69,6% expressed CD68), with a remaining 30,4% non CD68 expressing subjects, with eta coefficient was 0,647 (table 9). Only 8,7% of non endometriosis subjects expressed CD68 macrophage, with a IHC score of +1. Contradictively, all endometriosis subjects expressed CD163 macrophages, with the following incidence rates: 21,7%, 30,4%, and 47,8% subjects expressing +1, +2, and +3 CD 163 macrophages, respectively, the results of which are displayed in table 16. Whereas only 8,7% of non endometriosis subjects expressed CD163 macrophages.

Table 15 Association between CD68 macrophage expression and endometriosis

	IHC SCORE				r*	p**
	0	+1	+2	+3		
Endometriosis	7 (30,4%)	5 (21,7%)	6 (26,1%)	5 (21,7%)	0,647	0,001
Non endometriosis	21 (91,3%)	2 (8,7%)	0 (0%)	0 (0%)		

*Eta Correlation, **Chi-square test*

Table 16 Association between CD163 macrophage expression and endometriosis

	IHC SCORE				r*	p**
	0	+1	+2	+3		
Endometriosis	0 (0%)	5 (21,7%)	7 (30,4%)	11 (47,8%)	0,936	0,001
Non endometriosis	21 (91,3%)	2 (8,7%)	0 (0%)	0 (0%)		

*Eta Correlation, **Chi-square test*

Results from table 17 shows that macrophages from CD68 expressing endometriosis lesions significantly differ to their counterparts from CD163 expressing lesions, with positive CD68 and CD163 cell expressions of 34,783 ±28,939 and 60,870 ±18,194, respectively (p<0,0001). Alternatively, activated CD163 macrophages were more frequently encountered than CD68 counterparts Immunohistochemical testing reported that CD68 and CD163 macrophages infiltrate endometriosis lesions, although non endometriosis specimens also revealed similar findings.

Table 17 Macrophage positive cell percentages: a comparison in endometriosis

Marker	Mean Positive cells (±SD)	CI 95%	p*
CD68	34,783 (±28,939)	22,27 – 47,30	0,001
CD163	60,870 (±18,194)	53,00 – 68,74	

Independent sample t-test

CD68 expression did not significantly differ between degrees of severity (p-value 0,995, table 18). Expression of lesion infiltrating macrophages did not differ in moderate-severe cases, with 28,6%, 23,8%, 28,6% and 19% endometriosis subjects expressing CD68 IHC scores of 0, +1, +2, and +3, respectively. Mild-minimal degree subjects also showed a similar tendency. Although expression rates was increased in moderate-severe cases (23,8%, 28,6%, and 47,6% subjects expressed +1, +2 and +3 CD163), CD163 expression also did not significantly differ between degrees of endometriosis, as shown by results displayed in table 13 (p-value 1,0).

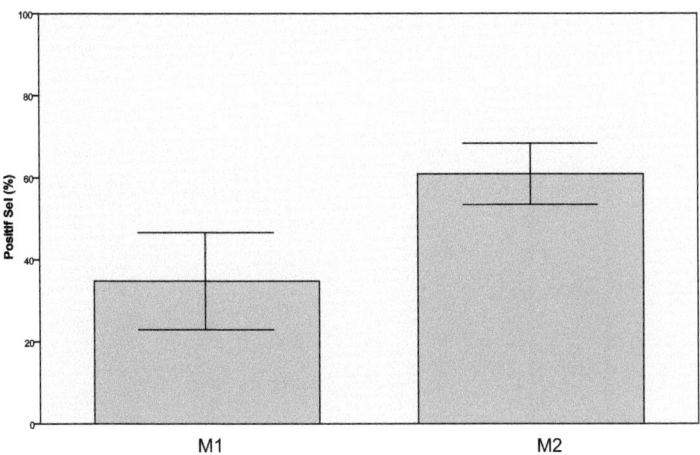

Graphic 1 Comparison of mean M1 (CD68) and M2 (CD163) positive cells in endometriosis

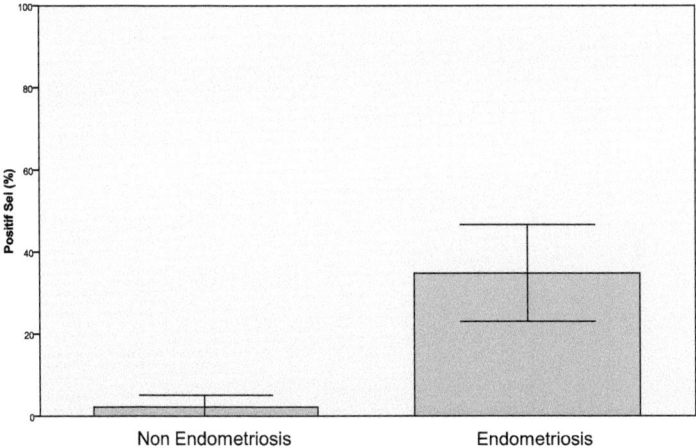

Graphic 2 Comparison of mean M1 (CD68) positive cells in Endometriosis dan Non Endometriosis specimens

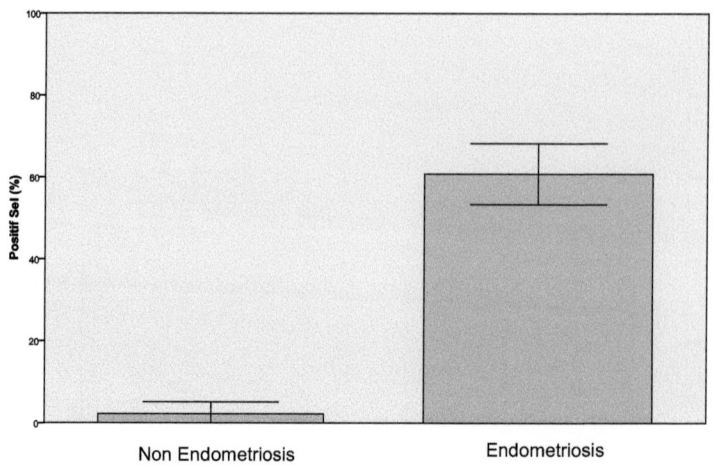

Graphic 3 Comparison of mean M2 (CD163) positive cells in Endometriosis dan Non Endometriosis specimens

Table 18 Association between severity degrees of endometriosis and CD68 expression

Severity degrees of Endometriosis	Immunohistochemical scoring of CD68				p*
	0	+1	+2	+3	
Minimal – Mild	1 (50%)	0 (0%)	0 (0%)	1 (50%)	0,995
Moderate – Severe	6 (28,6%)	5 (23,8%)	6 (28,6%)	4 (19%)	

Kolmogorov-Smirnov Z test

Table 19 Associaton between severity degrees of endometriosis expression of CD163

Severity degrees of Endometriosis	Immunohistochemical scoring of CD163			p*
	+1	+2	+3	
Minimal – Mild	0 (0%)	1 (50%)	1 (50%)	1,0
Moderate – Severe	5 (23,8%)	6 (28,6%)	10 (47,6%)	

Kolmogorov-Smirnov Z test

Table 20 displays that S allele containing (PS and SS) genotypes was encountered in 68% of CD163 macrophage expressing specimens, indicating that CD163 expression (M2) was significantly associated with certain genotypes (p-value 0,043).

Table 20 Association between L-selectin gene P213S polymorphism genotype on expression of CD163 and CD68

Genotype	Expression of CD163		p*	Expression of CD68		p*
	Positive CD163	Negative CD163		Positive CD68	Negative CD68	
PP	8 (38,1%)	13 (61,9%)	0,043	7 (33,3%)	14 (66,7%)	0,46
PS + SS	17 (68%)	8 (32%)		11 (44%)	14 (56%)	

*Chi-square test

However, contradictive results are shown, indicating that P213S genotypes of L-selectin genes were apparently not significantly associated with CD68 expression. CD68 was found positive in 33,33% and 44% of PP and PS+SS genotypes, respectively. The expression of CD 163 is displayed in figures 9 and 10.

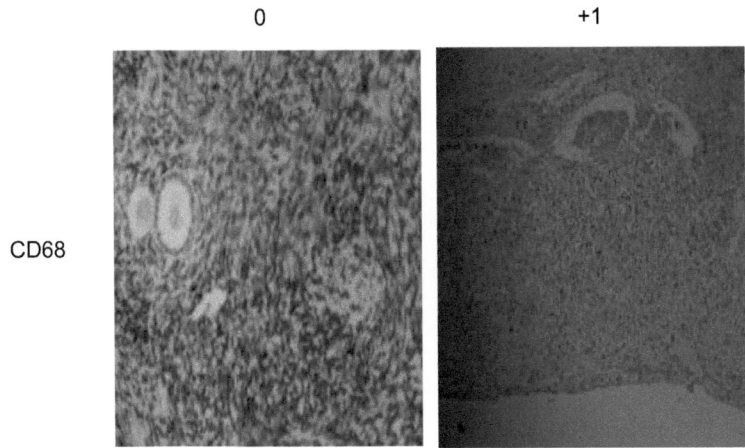

Figure 7. 0 and +1 CD 68 expression

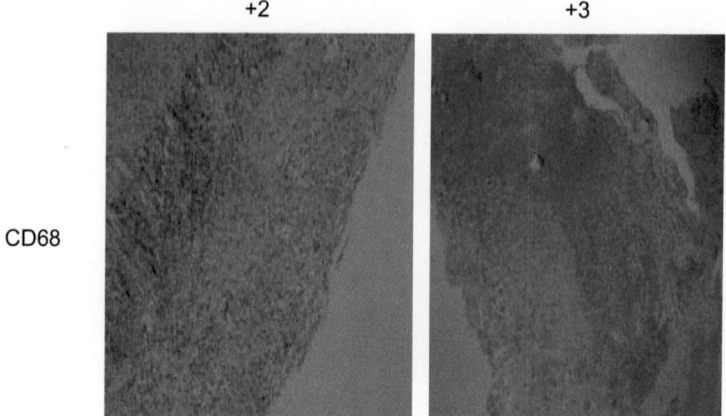

+2   +3

CD68

Figure 8. +2 and +3 CD 68 expression

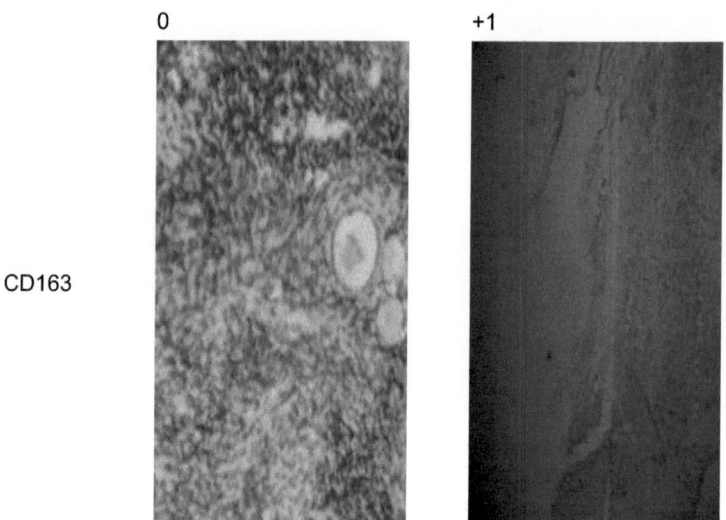

0   +1

CD163

Figure 9. 0 and +1 CD 163 expression

+2   +3

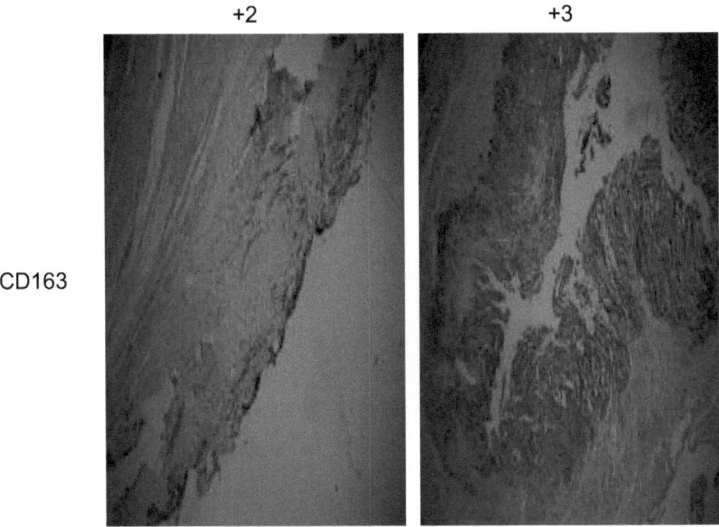

CD163

Figure 10. +2 and +3 CD 163 expression

Hypothesis Testing
Hypothesis I

Bivariate analysis shows that S allele subjects had a 2,893 (95% CI; 1,135-7,373) higher risk of developing endometriosis than P allele subjects, with a p value of 0,026 (p<0,05). Results also revealed that PS and SS genotyped subjects had a 3,556 higher risk of developing endometriosis than their PP genotyped counterparts (95% CI; 1,049-12, 052, with a p-value 0,041), thus indicating that L-selectin gene P213S polymorphism is associated with the incidence of endometriosis.

Hypothesis II

Analysis through differentiating average positive cells expressed from CD68 and CD163 antigenes (designated as M1 and M2 respectively) showed that CD163 was more frequently expressed than CD68, in endometriosis lesions (60,870 ±28,939 vs 34,783 ±18,194) with a p-value 0,0001. Positive immunohistochemical scorings revealed that CD68 macrophages was less frequently expressed (69,96%) than CD163 macrophages (100%) with a p-value 0,0001, indicating different roles of M1 and M2 macrophages in the pathogenesis of endometriosis.

Chapter 5
Discussion

Role of L-selectin gene p213s Polymorphism in Endometriosis

Predisposition to endometriosis include genes involved in molecular process that controls ectopic endometrial cell survival, and endometrial cell invasion to the peritoneal surface, proliferation, neovascularization, or inflammatory response. In women with endometriosis, cell adhesion molecule expression show abnormlities in the peritoneal eutopic endometrium (Tseng et al., 1996; Noblee et al., 1996; Fritz et al., 2011). Rat model transplantated with endometriosis tissues tevealed 45 gene expression encoding cytokinees, growth factors, and cell adhesion molecules associated with endometriosis. Among several genes with indistinct increase of osteopontin transcription, Lyn, Vav1, Runx1 and L-Selectin in endometriosis tissues compared to eutopic endometrium (Konno et al., 2007). However, no testing for gene polymorphism performed in humans has known to effect expression in several genes, including L-selectin, which was associated with endometriosis.

L-selectin is a glycoprotein adhesion cell located in the lymphocytes (Odagiri et al., 2007), the role of which is important in binding lymphocytes to high endothelial venules (HEV) (Paschall, 2007). L-selectin also plays an important role in the early steps of leukocyte recruitment from circulation to peripheral inflammatory sites including rolling leukocytes followed by activating leukocytes, significant adhesions, and leukocyte transmigration to interstitial tissue (Rosen SD, 2004; Hafezi-Moghadam, et al., 2001) subsequently affecting inflammatory substance secretion, including growth factors, chemokinees, cytokinee, complements, protease, nitric oxide, and reactive oxygen metabolite (Crockett-Torabi et al., 1996) that play a role in the pathogenesis of endometriosis. L-selectin gene polymorphism located in chromosome 1 in locus q23-q25 (Iida et al., 2003), has frequently been associated with several inflammatory associated diseases (Stavarachi et al, 2009). Several studies have shown that mutated single C nucleotides (Cytosine) are transformed into Timin in Graves's disease, Type 1 diabetes (Chen et al., 2007; Kretowski et al., 2000), resulting in altered biological activity effects of L-selectin genes.

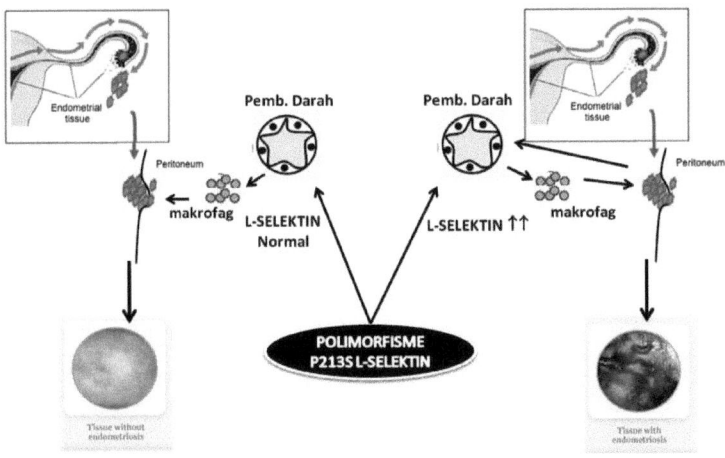

Figure 11. Role of L-selectin Polymorphism in Endometriosis

This study showed that S allele subjects (with L-selectin gene P213S polymorphismgene) have a 3 time higher risk than P allele subjects to develop endometriosis (OR 2,893; 95% CI; 1,135-7,373 with a p value 0,026). Appearance of S allele containing genotypes (PS and SS) indicated a 4 time higher risk than normal PP genotypes (OR 3,55; CI 95% 1,049 sampai 12,052) and confirmed findings by Konno et al, revealing that L-selectin gene trancriptions was more frequently found in endometriosis lesions than non-endometriosis specimens (Konno et al., 2007). This indicated that P213S polymorphism increased L-selectin transcription, that would then result in increased monocyte and macrophage recruitment to endometriosis lesions. As stated above, SNPs are the source of genomic variety. SNPs are various sources of a genom and are generally a mutated base form. They are the most simple and common form of human genetic polymorphism (Kaleigh, 2002). As they are located on regulator elements (such as gene promotors, enhancers or silencers) and coding regions, synonymous SNPs, may cause amino acid alterations, frame shifts or terminated translations, consequently providing functional effects on protein levels (Sundqvist, 2011). P213S polymorphism is itself an SNP, in which the 637th base is converted (from Cytosine to Thymine on exon 6), resulting in amino acid coding on codon 213 (from Proline to Serine). Exon 6 located on the L-selectin gene, is known as the domain of the Short Consensus Repeat (SCR1), that functions in cell adhesions, oligomerization, optimizes Epidermal Growth Factor (EGF) and lectin domains (Stavarachi et al, 2009). Consequently, exon polymorphism would affect L-selectin gene SCR1 associated functions. In this study, this event is stressed as mostly associated with the events of endometriosis.

Combining L- selectin with monoclonal antibodies and ligands may cause cellular morphological changes, changes in cellular action patterns, and increased IL-8 and increased TNF-α expressions (Chen et al., 2006; Crockett-Torabi et al., 1996). IL-8 is known to increase in peritoneal washings of women with endometriosis and correlates with the severity of the disease, and may also act as endometrial autocrine growth factors. Therfore, IL-8 may affect endometrial cell and cell growth. TNF-α is a product of activated macrophages that activate leukocytes during inflamation and direct production other proinflammatory cytokinees, including IL-1 IL-6, dan TNF-α. These cytokines stimulate endometrial cellular adhesion, induce MMP expression, and affect ectopic endometrial tissue implantation to the peritoneum (Eisenberg et al., 2012).

This study shows that PS and SS genotypes are more significantly associated with the events of endometriosis (69,6%) than PP genotyped specimens PP (30,4%) (p = 0,038), whereas no non endometriosis subject was SS genotyped. S alleles was more frequently encountered in endometriosis specimens than the control group (41,3% vs 19,6% dengan p = 0,023).

As endometriosis is affected by various factors, including hormones, enviromental exposure (dioxyn), and genetics, P and S alleles were weakly correlated with the events of endometriosis. Presence of P alleles does not not automatically designate inability for endometriosis, and contradictively, S allele women do not indicate otherwise. This is evidently shown by an OR value of 2.893 for S alleles to develop endometriosis. A study by Odagiri et al shows that in cases of human endometriosis, L-selectin was expressed in tissue lymphocyte cells and macrophages and on immunohistochemically testing eutopic endometrium, no L-selectin expression was observed (Odagiri et al., 2007). Leukocyte located L-selectins would only be activated during an inflammatory process through the presence of chemokinee, such as MCP-1 and RANTES produced by ectopic endometrial cells, subsequently increasing monocyte and macrophage recruitment in to endometriosis tissues (Hornung, et. al., 2001; Nasu et. al., 2007), therefore indicating that L-selectin was clearly expressed in endometriosis lesions. In a rat model, endometriosis tissues was observed with a 46 time L-selectin mRNA transciption increase normal endometrium specimens (Konno et al., 2007).

However, this study demonstrated that severity degrees of endometriosis were not associated with L-selectin gene P213S polymorphism. Prolonged presence of macrophages indicates chronic inflammation through formation of granulation tissues by necrosis, encapsulating fibrosis, and/or several degrees of scar tissue formation (Anderson et al., 2008; Ratner BD, 2004; Valentine, 2003). Altrnative macrophages and circulating monocytes in women with enometriosis seem to support endometriosis by secreting growth factors and cytokinees, stimulating ectopic endometrial proliferation including IL-8, IL-6, TNF-α, IL-22 and inhibiting scavenging functions (Ilie et al., 2013; Murdoch et al., 2004; Coussens et al., 2000; Fritz et al., 2011). Severity degrees of endometriosis are based on pelvic organ involvement, whereas extent of attachment is affected by several factors. Inflammatory process triggers cytokinee and growth factor expressions, from which macrophages stimulate fibrosis formation through myelofibroblast collagens resulting in enhanced adhesions (Wynn et al., 2010; Matalliotakis et al., 2003). However, as reported by Tempfer et al, endomeriosis may affect several gen polymorphisms, that apart from inflammatory process and cellular adhesion, are also associated with hormonal biosynthesis, growth factor genes, etc (Tempfer et al., 2009).

Other studies associated with L-selectin inhibiting therapies in endometriosis have yet to be reported. However, a study by Asimakopoulus et al., 2000 reported the use of aprotinin to obtain anti-inflammatory potency by inhibiting neutrophil L-selectin cardiopulmonary bypass (Asimakopoulos et al., 2000).

M1 and M2 Macrophage profiles in Endometriosis

Peritoneal macrophage count and activation status increase in women with endometriosis. Increased growth factors and cytokinees affect survival and endometriosis cellular growth, and may cause receptor functional disability. Activating macrophages, through cytokine and growth factor release, may contribute to the coinciding early formation and development of endometriosis (Eisenberg et al., 2012). Monocyte/macrophage recruitment and activation may induce local inflammatory reactions and is highly affected by excessive expressions of macrophage activating factors mainly produced by eutopic endometrial cells, including MCP-1, makrofag *migration inhibitory factors* (MIF) dan IL-1(Ilie et al., 2013).

Macrophages functions by regulating anti tumor immunity responses. In the presence of stromal remodelling-associated tumor growth factors and proinflammatory molecule production as foreign bodies, M1 macrophages, like NK cells (Oosterlynck et al., 1991; Oosterlynck et al., 1992), produce IFN-γ and IL-12 secretion-mediated responses (Tsung et al., 2002; Brigati et al., 2002). On activating IFN-γ, M1 would release tumoricidal products including, reactive oxygen intermediates and nitric oxide, that function as tumor cell destroyers (MacMiking et al., 1997). These activated macrophages subsequently produce TNF-α, consequently destroying foreign bodies by inhibiting vascular formation (Blankenstein et al., 1991).

Cytokine production (IL-8, IL-6, TNF-α, IL-22) (Ilie et al., 2013) may stimulate endothelial cellular proliferation and angiogenesis in the presence of M2 macrophages (Murdoch et al., 2004; Coussens et al., 2000). Studies on experimental rats show that alternatively activated macrophages (M2 macrophages) dramatically increase endometriosis lesions in rat, whereas inflammatory macrophages (M1 macrophages) effectively protect rats from endometriosis. Therefore, M2 macrophages involved in tissue remodelling seem, to affect the natural course of endometriosis, necessitating effective vasular formation and growth of endometriosis lesions (Martinez et al., 2008; Bacci et al., 2009).

Alternatively activating macrophages (M2 macrophages) is a key step in the development of endometriosis, in which increased M2 macrophages would secrete and enhance cytokines, prostaglandins, components, and growth factors (tumor necrosis factor-β (TNF-α), IL-6, and transforming growth factor-β (TGF-β)) concentrations. Normally, endometriosis cells entering the peritoneal cavity are eliminated by macrophages. Aberrations in endometriosis result in an ineffective immunological cearing system to foreign bodies. Apart from neovascularization, M2 macrophages and increased levels of cytokines also result in endometrial cell initiation, progression, and growth (Gupta et al, 2006). IL-22 is known to affect release of several chemokines, including CXCL1, CXCL5, CXCL9, and CCL2. CCL2, CXCR1 and IL-8 are konwn to regulate endometrial stromal cells and is therefore associated with growth of endometriosis cells (Ilie et al., 2013). M2 macrophages therefore tend to positively effect on cellular or tumor growth.

As a result, M2 macrophages have been evidently shown to have a more significant role than M1 macrophages in the pathogenesis of endonetriosis. This may be due to genetic, hormonal and enviromental factors. A study reported that estrogen increased M2 macrophage activities through estrogen receptors expressed by surface macrophages. Under estrogen control, M2 macrophages secrete cytokines and growth factors (including VEGF, hepatocyte growth factor, dan TNF-α) contributing to the development and persistance of endometriosis (Gordon S, 2007; Montagna et al., 2008).

From several inflammatory mediators involved in endometriosis, RANTES, a specific chemokine, was also increased. RANTES was synthesized and secreted by endometriosis cells whereas monocyte cells express RANTES receptors including CCR1 and CCR5 consequently causing chemotactic stiumlation resulting in peritoneal leukocyte infiltration. TNF-α dan IFN-γ would also increase expression from these chemokine receptors. In vitro studies reported that stimulating endometrial cells using TNF-α dan IFN-γ increased RANTES mRNA protein expressions (Khorram et al., 1993; Hornung, et. al., 2001; Nishida et al., 2011). RANTES is known to cause 70% of migrating monocytes to peritoneal washings of endometriosis patients (Hornung et al., 2001).

MCP-1 also facilitates macrophage activation through CCR2 and CCR4. MCP-1, produced endometrial epithelial and stromal cells (Arici et al., 1995; Jones et al., 1997; Jolicoeur et al., 1998) is affected by estradiol and progesterone and also by IL-13 (Nasu et al., 2003), TNF-β (Arici et al., 1995; Nasu et al., 2003), IFN-α (Arici et al., 1995), IFN-γ (Nasu et al., 1998), IL-1β (Kang et al., 2004), consequently increasing monocyte and macrophage recruitment and activation (Nasu et. al., 2007). Local estrogen levels are known to increase through aromatase reactions in endometriosis lesions consequently enhancing chemokine production by endometrial cells that eavantually affects monocyte and macrophage recruitment (Akoum et al., 2000). Valesco et al cultured endometriosis tissues and found significant aromatase expressions in these specimens and no expression of P450 aromatase in normal endometrial tissues (Valesco et al., 2006).

This study reported that M1 macrophage (CD68) and M2 macrophages (CD163) significantly differed. M2 macrophages were more highly expressed than M1 macrophages in endometriosis lesions. Increased macrophage activation, together with increased secretion and synthesis of several proinflammatory mendiators, such as cytokinees, are known to occur in endometriosis lesions than non endometriosis normal peritoneum (Taylor et al. 1997). M1 macrophages was observed in eutopic endometrium of women diagnosed with endometriosis with various levels in each menstrual phase. M1 macrophages were also increased in eutopic endometrum women with endometriosis encountered during the proliferative phase (Berbic et al. 2009). A study on rat models using endometriosis transplantation reported increased macrophage markers with various expression intensities and reported similar results, in which M2 macrophages were more highly expressed than M1 macrophages in endometriosis lesions. Immunohistochemical testing revealed that M1 macrophages infiltrates endometriosis lesions, however, these macrophages are also present in the non endometriosis peritoneum. M2 macrophages were only observed in endometriosis lesions (Bacci et al., 2009).

Normal mentruation is affected by estrogen and progesteron that stimulate endometrial cells to produce chemokines, including MCP-1 and RANTES. These chemokines would subsequently trigger an inflammatory process resulting in macrophage recruitment, activated clasically (M1) or alternatively (M2). This sequence would take place normally, following the menstrual cycle (Bacci et al., 2009; Thiruchelvam et al., 2013). This study shows differed expressions of M1 and M2 macrophages, with significantly higher M2 macrophage expressions in endometriosis. M2 macrophages had a stronger correlation than M1 macrophages with correlation eta coefficients of 0.9 and 0.6 for M2 and M1, respectively, in cases of endometriosis.

This study showed that CD68 was more highly expressed in endometriosis tissues than non endometriosis tissues. Similar results by Tran et al reported higher CD 68 expressions in endometriosis lesions than non endometriosis peritoneal macrophages (Tran et al., 2009). As previously stated, M1 macrophages comply to the normal inflammatory process and is constantly balanced by M2 macrophage counterparts. Bacci et al also stated that CD163 was more higly expressed in endometriosis lesions than non endometriosis specimens.

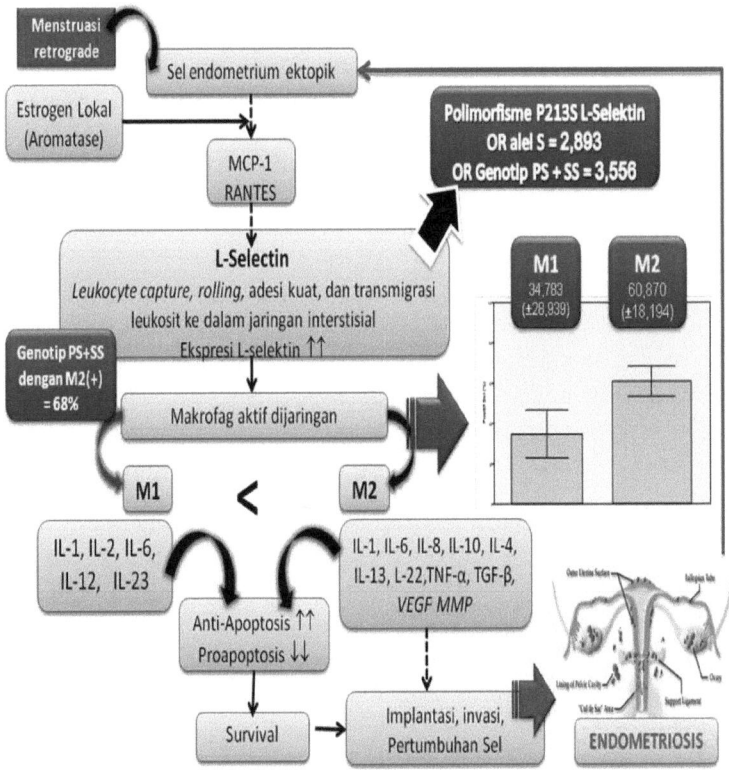

Figure 12. Role of L-selectin polymorphism in L-selectin and Macrophage profiles in Endometriosis

These results together with findings from other studies and pathogenesis theories of endometriosis are described in the image above. Almost every woman experience retrograde menstruation each month. Physiologically, each endometrial cell would cause an inflammatory reaction by producing MC-1 and RANTES from stromal cells and endometrial glands triggered by estrogen produced by the aromatase process. This chemokine also affects monocyte and macrophage recruitment to endometriosis lesions. However, the main issue remains as to, although most women experience retrograde menstruation, why do only 5 to 10% of them experience endometriosis. Patients with endometriosis are presented with altered inflammatory balances, apoptosis process, triggered by genetic polymorphism, including L-selectin. As previously explained, L-selectin polymorphism plays a signifcant role in this matter, causing increased monocyte and M1 macrophage recruitments into endometriosis lesions to trigger apoptosis, cytotoxic and phagocytosis, by secreting certain cytokinees. These also include cytokinees produced by M2 macrophages that trigger cellular growth and repair. However, due to changes in biological effects as a result of L-selectin P213S ploymoprhism evidently shown by significant L-selectin expressions in endometriosis tissues, M2 apparently is more dominantly activated than M1. The apoptosis process is subsequently compromised, with surviving cells consequently increasing the inflammatory process by recruiting macrophages. Facilitated by adhesive cells, surviving endometriosis cells would then undergo implantation, causing endometriosis cell growth and development. These facts support the motion that M1 and M2 imbalance in patients with endometriosis is triggered by L-selectin polymorphism.

Chapter 6
Conclusions and Recommendations

Conclusions

L-selectin gene P213 S polymorphism affects the events of endometriosis. S alleles are more frequently encountered in the endometriosis group than non-endometriosis group (41,3% vs 19,6%) with a p value of 0,023. S allele genotypes (PS and SS) were also more frequently found in the former group than the latter (69,6% vs 39,1%) as were they more frequently encountered than P alleles in the endometriosis group (69,6% vs 30,4%).

L-selectin gene P213S polymorphism was associated with the events of endometriosis. Bivariate analysis showed that S alleles have a 2,893 higher risk (CI 95% 1,135 to 7,373, p = 0,026) for endometriosis than P alleles. Comparison between genotypes PS and SS with PP showed a 3,556 higher risk for developing endometriosis in the former group than the latter (CI 95% 1,049 to 12, 052, p value of 0,041).

M2 macrophages are significantly more involved than M1 macrophages in the pathogenesis of endometriosis, with higher expressions of CD163 than CD68 (60,870 ±28,939 vs 34,783 ±18,194 with p value of 0,0001). Positive immunohistochemical scoring showed that 69,6% and 100% of endometriosis lesion expressed CD 68 and CD163, respectively (p value 0.0001).

Recommendation

On confirming the role it has on the events of endometriosis, L-selectin gene is expected to be a marker in diagnosing this disease. Measures to prevent development of ectopic endometrial cells are therefore possible in women with L-selectin gen S allele polymorphism. Further studies concerning L-selectin targeted therapies are neccessary in attempt to prevent the events of endometriosis. In unprevented cases, these further studies could be used to effectively treat endometriosis.

Intervention through recovering inflammatory factors associated with the events of endometriosis, including the association with role of macrophages and other inflammatory mediators, should also be futher studies. Methods to covert M2 macrophages into M1 macrophages should also be sought.

References

Akoum A, Jolicoeur C, Boucher A. 2000. Estradiol amplifies iinterleukin-1 induced monocyte chemotactic protein-1 expression by ectopic endometrial cells of women with endometriosis. J Clin Endocrinol Metab. 85: 896-904

Allavena P, Sica A, Solinas G, Porta C, Mantovani A. 2008. The inflammatory micro-environment in tumor progression: the role of tumor-associated macrophages. Crit Rev Oncol Hematol. 66(1):1-9

Altshuler, D., Daly, M. J. and Lander, E. S. 2008. Genetic mapping in human disease. Science, 322, 881-888.

Anderson JM, Rodriguez A, Chang DT. 2008. Foreign body reaction to biomaterials. Semin Immunol. Apr;20(2):86-100.

Arici A, MacDonald P, casey ML. 1995. Regulation of manocyte chometactic protein-1 gene expression in human endometrial cells in cultures. Mol Cell Endocrinol. 94: 195-204

Arrive L, Hricak H, Martin MC, 1989. Pelvic endometriosis: MR imaging, Radiology 171:687.

Asimakopoulos G, Taylor KM, Haskard DO, Landis RC. 2000. Inhibition of neutrophil L-selectin shedding: a potential anti-inflammatory effect of aprotinin. Perfusion. 15(6):495-9.

Bacci, M., Capobianco, A., Monno, A., Cottone, L., Di Puppo, F., Camisa, B., et al., 2009. Macrophages Are Alternatively Activated in Patients with Endometriosis and Required for Growth and Vascularization of Lesions in a Mouse Model of Disease. Am J Pathol. 175(2):547-556

Badylak, S.F., Valentin, J.E., Ravindra, A.K., McCabe, G.P., and Stewart-Akers, A.M., 2008. Macrophage Phenotype as a Determinant of Biologic Scaffold Remodeling. Tissue Engineering Part A. 14(11): 1835-1842

Balasch J, Creus M, Fabregeus F, et al. 1996. Visible and nonâ€"visible endometriosis at laparoscopy in fertile and infertile women and in patients with chronic pelvic pain: a prospective study. Hum Reprod; 11:387-391.

Baziad, A., 2008. Endokrinologi Ginekologi: Endometriosis . Edisi ketiga. Jakarta. Penerbit Media Aesculapius. Fakultas Kedokteran Universitas Indonesia: 1-31

Bazot M, Malzy P, Cortez A, Roseau G, Amouyal P, Darai E, 2007. Accuracy of transvaginal sonography and rectal endoscopic sonography in the diagnosis of deep infiltrating endometriosis, Ultrasound Obstet Gynecol 30:994.

Berbic, M., and Fraser, I.S., 2011. Regulatory T cells and other leukocytes in the pathogenesis of endometriosis. J Reprod Immunol. 88(2): 149-155

Berbic, M., Schuke, L., Markham, R., Tokushige, N., Russell, P., and Fraser, I.S., 2009. Macrophage expression in endometrium of women with and without endometriosis. Hum Reprod. 241(2): 325-332

Blankenstein, T., Qin, Z., Uberla, K., Muller, W,., Rosen, H., Volk, H., et al. 1991. Tumor Suppression after tumor cell targeted tumor necrosis factor α gene transfer. J Exp Med. 173(5): 1047-1052

Brigati, C., Noonan, D.M., Albini, A., Benelli, R., 2002. Tumors and inflammatory infiltrates : friends od foes? Clin Exp Metastasis. 19(3): 247-258

Buelke SJ, Bryant HU, Francis PC. 1998. The selective estrogen receptor modulator, raloxifene: an overview of nonclinical pharmacology and reproductive and developmental testing. Reprod Toxicol;12:217-221.

Bulun, S.E., 2009. Mechanism of Disease Endometriosis. N Eng J Med. 360(3): 268-279.

Carr, B.R., 2008. Chapter 10 : Endometriosis. In: Schorge, J.O., Schaffer, J.I., Halvorson, L.M., Hoffman, B.L., Bradshaw, K.D., Cunningham, F.G., William's Gynecology. McGraw-Hill Company.

Chapron C, Fauconnier A, Dubuisson JB, et al. 2003. Deep infiltrating endometriosis: relation between severity of dysmenorrhoea and extent of disease. Hum Reprod;18:760-766

Chatman DL, Ward AB, 1982. Endometriosis in adolescents, J Reprod Med 27:156.

Chen, C., Ba, X., Xu, T., Cui, L., Hao, S., and Zeng, X., 2006. c-Abl is involved in the F-actin assembly triggered by L-selectin crosslinking. J Biochem. 140(2): 229–235

Chen, H.Y., Cui, B., Wang, S., Zhao, Z.F., Sun, H., Zhoa, Y.J., et al. 2007. L-selectin gene polymorphisms in Graves' disease. Clin Endocrinol (Oxf). 67(1): 145–151

Corna G, Campana L, Pignatti E, Castiglioni A, Tagliafico E, et al., 2010. Polarization dictates iron handling by inflammatory and alternatively activated macrophages. Haematologica.95(11):1814-1822

Cornillie FJ, Oosterlynck D, Lauweryns JM, et al. 1990.Deeply infiltrating pelvic endometriosis: histology and clinical significance. Fertil Steril.;53:978-983

Coussens, L.M., Tinkle, C.L., Hanahan, D., and Werb, Z., 2000. MMP-9 supplied by bone marrow-derived cells contributes to skin carcinogenesis. Cell. 103(3): 481-490

Cramer DW, Wilson E, Stillman RJ, Berger MJ, Belisle S, Schiff I, Albrecht B, Gibson M, Stadel BV, Schoenbaum SC, 1986. The relation of endometriosis to menstrual characteristics, smoking and exercise, JAMA 355:1904.

Cramer, D.W., and Missmer, S.A., 2002. The epidemiology of endometriosis. Ann NY Acad Sci. 955: 11-22, discussion 34-6, 396-406

Crockett-Torabi, E., and Ward, P.A., 1996. The Role of Leukocytes in tissue injury. European Journal of Anaesthesiology. 13(3): 235-246

D'Hooghe, T.M., and Hill, J.A., 2007. Endometriosis. In: Berek, J.S., Berek & Novak's Gynecology. 14th Edition. Philadelphia. Lippincott Williams & Wilkin: 1137-84

Daly, M. J., Rioux, J. D., Schaffner, S. F., Hudson, T. J. and Lander, E. S. 2001. Highresolution haplotype structure in the human genome. Nat Genet, 29, 229-232.

Darya HR, Siregar HS, et al., 2014. Perbedaan IL-2 pada wanita penderita endometriosis dan wanita non endometriosis. Universitas Sumatera Utara. Medan.

D'Hooghe TM, Bambra CS, Raeymaekers BM, De Jonge I, Lauweryns JM, Koninckx PR, 1995. Intrapelvic injection of menstrual endometrium causes endometriosis in baboons (Papio cynocephalus and Papio anubis), Am J Obstet Gynecol 173:125.

D'Hooghe TM, Nugent N, Cuneo S, et al. 2006. Recombinant human TNF binding protein inhibits the development of endometriosis in baboons: a prospective, randomized, placebo and drug controlled study. Biology of Reproduction;74:131-136.

Eisenberg, V.H., Zolti, M., and Soriano, D., 2012. Is There an assosiation between autoimmunity and endometriosis?. Autoimmunity Reviews. 11: 806-814

Eskenazi, B., and Warner, M.G.,1997. Epidemiology of endometriosis. Obstet Gynecol Clin North Am, 24 (2): 235-258

Fahmi MF, Adenin I, Siregar HS, et al., 2014. Kadar Vascular Endothelial Growth Factor (VEGF) serum pada wanita dengan endometriosis. Universitas Sumatera Utara. Medan.

Falconer, H., Mwenda, J. M., Chai, D. C., Wagner, C., Song, X. Y., Mihalyi, A., Simsa, P., Kyama, C., Cornillie, F. J., Bergqvist, A. et al. 2006. Treatment with anti-TNF monoclonal antibody (c5N) reduces the extent of induced endometriosis in the baboon. Hum Reprod, 21, 1856-1862.

Fauconnier A, Chapron C, Dubuisson JB, et al. 2002. Relation between pain symptoms and the anatomic location of deep infiltrating endometriosis. Fertil Steril;78(4):719-726.

Frazer, K. A., Murray, S. S., Schork, N. J. and Topol, E. J. 2009. Human genetic variation and its contribution to complex traits. Nat Rev Genet, 10, 241-251.

Fritz, M.A., and Speroff, L., 2011. Clinical Gynecologic Endocrinology and Infertility: Endometriosis. 8th edition. Lippincott Williams & Wilkins. North Caroline:1103-25

Goldstein DP, deCholnoky C, Emans SJ, Leventhal JM, 1989.Laparoscopy in the diagnosis and management of pelvic pain in adolescents, J Reprod Med 24:251.

Gordon S. 2007. The macrophage: past, present and future. Eur J Immunol. 37 (1):S9-17.

Gupta, S., Agarwal, A., Sekhon, L., Krajcir, N., Cocuzza, M., and Falcone, T., 2006. Serum and Peritoneal Abnormalities in Endometriosis: Potential Use As Diagnostic Markers. Minerva Ginecol. 58(6):527-551

Hafezi-Moghadam, A., Thomas, K.L., Prorock, A.J., Huo, Y., and Ley, K., 2001. L-selectin shedding regulates leukocyte recrutment. J. Exp. Med. 193(7): 863-872

Hajilooi, M., Tajik, N., Sanati, A., Eftekhari, H., Massoud, A., 2006. Association of the Phe206Leu allele of the L-Selectin gene with coronary artery disease. Cardiology. 105(2):113-138

Halme J, Hammond MG, Hulka JF, Raj SG, Talbert LM, 1984. Retrograde menstruation in healthy women and in patients with endometriosis, Obstet Gynecol 64:151.

Hediger ML, Hartnett HJ, Louis GM, 2005Association of endometrio sis with body size and figure, Fertil Steril 84:1366

Hesla, J.S., and Rock, J.A., 2008. Chapter 25 : Endometriosis. In: Rock, J.A., Jones, H.W., Te Linde's Operative Gynecology. Tenth Edition. Philadephia. Lippincott Williams & Wilkins. 245-254.

Hornung, D,, Bentzien, F., Wallwiener, D., Kiesel, L., Taylor, R.N., 2001. Chemokinee bioactivity of RANTES in endometriotic and normal endometrial stromal cells and peritoneal fluid. Molecular Human Reproduction. 7(2): 163-168

Hummelshoj, L., Prentice, A., and Groothuis, P., 2006. Update on endometriosis. Women Health (Lond Engl). 2(1): 53-56

Iida, A., and Nakamura, Y., 2003. High-resolution SNP map in the 55-kb region containing the selectin gene family on chromosome 1q24–q25. J Hum Genet. 48(3):150–154

Ilie, I., and Ilie, R., 2013. Cytokinees and Endometriosis – the Role of Immunological Alterations. Biothecnology, Molecular biology and Nanomedicine. 1(2): 8-19

Jones RL, Kelly RW, Crtchley HOD. 1997. Chemokinee and cyclooxygenase-2 expression in human endometrium coincides with leukocyte accumulation. Hum Reprod. 12;1300-1306.

Jones, G., Jenkinson, C., and Kennedy, S., 2004. The impact of endometriosis upon quality of life: a qualitative analysis. J Psychosom Obstet Gynaecol, 25(2): 123-133

Kaleigh, S., 2002. Genetic Polymorphism and SNPs. 14(21)

Kaur, G., Rapthap, C.C., Kumar, S., Bhatnagar, S., Bhan, M.K., and Mehra, N.K., 2006. Polymorphism in L-selectin, E-selectin and ICAM-1 Genes in Asian Indian Pediatric Patients With Celiac Disease. Hum Immunol. 67(8): 634-638

Khazen, D., Jendoubi-Ayed, S., Aleya, W.B., Sfar, I., Mouelhi, L., Matri, S., et al. 2009. Polymorphism in ICAM-1, PECAM-1, E-selectin, and L-selectin gene in Tunisian patients with inflammatory bowel disease. European Journal Of Gastroenterology & Hepatology. 21(2):167-175

Khorram, O., Taylor, R. N., Ryan, I. P., Schall, T. J. and Landers, D. V. 1993. Peritoneal fluid concentrations of the cytokinee RANTES correlate with the severity of endometriosis. Am J Obstet Gynecol, 169, 1545-1549.

Koninckx PR, Meuleman C, Demeyere S, et al. 1991.Suggestive evidence that pelvic endometriosis is a progressive disease, whereas deeply infiltrating endometriosis is associated with pelvic pain. Fertil Steril;55:759-765

Koninckx PR, Meuleman C, Oosterlynck D, Cornillie FJ, 1996. Diagnosis of deep endometriosis by clinical examination during menstruation and plasma CA-125 concentration, Fertil Steril 65:280.

Konno, R., Fujiwara, H., Netsu, S., Odagiri, K., Shimane, M., Nomura, H., et al. 2007. Gene expression profiling of rat endometriosis model. Am J Reprod Immunol 58(4): 330-343

Kretowski, A., and Kinalska, I., 2000. L-selectin gene T668C mutation in type 1 diabetes patients and their first degree relatives. Immunol. Lett. 74(3): 225–228

Kuohung W, Jones GL, Vitonis AF, Cramer DW, Kennedy SH, Thomas D, Hornstein MD, 2002. Characteristics of patients with endometriosis in the United States and the United Kingdom, Fertil Steril 78:767.

Lebovic, D. I., Mueller, M. D. and Taylor, R. N. 2001. Immunobiology of endometriosis. Fertil Steril, 75, 1-10.

Ley, K., 2003. The role of selectins in inflammation and disease. TRENDS in Molecular Medicine. Elsevier. 9 (6): 263-268

Liu DTY, Hitchhock A, 1986. Endometriosis: its association with retrograde menstruation, dysmenorrhea, and tubal pathology, Br J Obstet Gynaecol 93:859.

Liu J., Liu, Jx., Xu, S., Quan, J., Tian, L., Guo, Q., 2012. Association of P213S polymorphism of the L-Selectin gene with type 2 diabetes and insulin resistance in chinese population. Gene. 509:286-290

Lorençatto, C., Petta, C.A., Navarro, M.J., Bahamondes, L., and Matos, A., 2006. Depression in women with endometriosis with and without chronic pelvic pain. Acta Obstet Gynecol Scand. 85(1): 88-92

MacMiking, J., Xie, Q.W., and Nathan, C., 1997. Nitric Oxide and macrophage function. Annu Rev Immunol. 15(1): 323-350

Mahmood TA, Templeton AA, Thomson L, Fraser C, 1991. Menstrual symptoms in women with pelvic endometriosis, Br J Obstet Gynaecol 98:558.

Manurung ES, Siregar HS, Nasution SA. 2013. Perbedaan Ekspresi Imunohistokimia Aromatase P450 Pada Endometrium Ektopik Penderita Endometriosis Dibandingkan dengan Endometrium Normal. Universitas Sumatera Utara. Medan.

Margarit L, Gonzalez D, Lewis PD, Hopkins L, Davies C, et al., 2009. L-Selectin ligands in human endometrium: comparison of fertile and infertile subjects. Hum Reprod. 24(11):2767-2777

Marpaung K, et al. 2013. Perbedaan kadar sL-Selectin pada wanita dengan endometriosis dibandingkan dengan non endometriosis. Universitas Sumatera Utara. Medan

Martinez FO, Sica A, Mantovani A, Locati M. 2008. Macrophage activation and polarization. Front Biosci. 13:453-61.

Matalliotakis IM, Goumenou AG, Koumantakis GE, Neonaki MA, Koumantakis EE, et al. 2003. Serum concentration of growth factors in women with and without endometriosis: the action of anti-endometriosis medicines. Int Immunopharmacol.3(1): p. 81-89.

Matarese, G., De Placido, G., Nikas, Y. and Alviggi, C. 2003. Pathogenesis of endometriosis: natural immunity dysfunction or autoimmune disease? Trends Mol Med, 9, 223-228.

Matorras R, Rodriguez F, Pijoan JI, Soto E, Perez C, Ramon O, Rodriguez-Escudero F, 1996. Are there any clinical signs and symptoms that are related to endometriosis in infertile women?, Am J Obstet Gynecol 174:620.

Missmer SA, Hankinson SE, Spiegelman D, Barbieri RL, Marshall LM, Hunter DJ, 2004. Incidence of laparoscopically confirmed endometriosis by demographic, anthropometric, and lifestyle factors, Am J Epidemiol 160:784.

Missmer SA, Hankinson SE, Spiegelman D, Barbieri RL, Michels KB, Hunter DJ, 2004. In utero exposures and the incidence of endometriosis, Fertil Steril 82:1501.

Montagna, P., Capellino, S., Villaggio, B., Remorgida, V., Ragni, N., Cutolo, M., et al., 2008. Peritoneal Fluid Macrophage in Endometriosis: Correlation Between The Expression Of Estrogen Receptors and Inflammation. Fertil Steril. 90(1): 156-164

Murdoch, C., Giannoudis, A., and Lewis, C.E., 2004. Mechanisms regulationg the recruitment of macrophages into hypoxic areas of tumor and other ischemic tissue. Blood. 104(8): 2224-2234

Nasu K, Fukuda J, Sun B, Nishida M, Miyakawa I. 2003. Interleukin-13 and tumor necrosis factor-β differentially regulate the production of cytokinee by cultured human endometrial stromal cells. Fertil Steril. 79(1);821-827

Nasu K, Matsui N, Narahara H, Tanaka Y, Miyakawa I. 1998. Effects of interferon-γ on cytokinee production by endometrial stromal cells. Hum reprod. 13;2598-2601

Nasu, K., Nishida, M., Yuge, A., and Narahara, H., 2007. Chapter 1: The Role of Chemokinee in the Pathogenesis of Endometriosis. In:Linkes WP, Progress in Chemokinee research. New York. Nova Science Publisher: 5-33

Nasution HHD, Siregar HS, Halim B, et al. 2013, 'Ekspresi L-Selectin pada Jaringan Endometriosis', Unversitas Sumatera Utara, Universitas Sumatera Utara, Medan.

Nezhat F, Allan CJ, Nezhat F, et al. 1991. Nonvisualized endometriosis at laparoscopy. Int J Fertil;36:340-343.

Nisolle M, Paindaveine B, Bourdin A, et al. 1990. Histological study of peritoneal endometriosis in infertile women. Fertil Steril;53:984-988.

Noble LS, Simpson ER, Johns A, Bulun SE. 1996. Aromatase expression in endometriosis. J Clin Endocrinol Metab; 81:174-9.

Noble LS, Takayama K, Zeitoun KM, et al. 1997. Prostaglandin E2 stimulates aromatase expression in endometriosis-derived stromal cells. J Clin Endocrinol Metab;82:600-6.

Noblee, A.D., and Lechworth, A.T. 1980. Treatment of Endometriosis: a study of management. Br J Obstet Gynecol. 87(8): 726-728

Oda, T., Katori, M., Hatanaka, K., and Yamashina, S., 1992. Five Steps in Leukocyte Extravasation in the Microcirculation by Chemoattractants. Yamagata University. Mediator of Inflammation. 1(6): 403-409

Odagiri, K., Konno, R., Fujiwara, H., Netsu, S., Ohwasa, M., Shibahara, H., et al. 2007. Immunohistochemical study of osteopontin (OPN) and L-selectin (SELL) in a rat endometriosis model and human endometriosis. Fertil Steril. 88(4 Suppl):1207-11

Oosterlynck DJ, Cornillie FJ, Waer M, Vandeputte M, Koninckx PR, 1991. Women with endometriosis show a defect in natural killer activity resulting in a decreased cytotoxicity to autologous endometrium, Fertil Steril 56:45.

Oosterlynck DJ, Meuleman C, Waer M, Vandeputte M, Koninckx PR, 1992. The natural killer activity of peritoneal fluid lymphocytes is decreased in women with endometriosis, Fertil Steril 58:292.

Osuga, Y., Koga, K., Hirota, Y., Hirata, T., Yoshino, O., and Taketani, Y., 2011. Lymphocytes in Endometriosis. Am J Reprod Immunol. 65(1): 1-10

Paschall, C.D., 2007. Cellular and Molecular Determinants of The L-selectin Shear Thresold Phenomenon. [Dissertation]. Virginia. University of Virginia.

Paul, D.W., and Braun, D.P., 2004. Immunology of endometriosis. Best Pract Res Clin Obstet Gynaecol. Elsevier. 18 (2):245-246

Pizzo, A., Salmeri, F. M., Ardita, F. V., Sofo, V., Tripepi, M. and Marsico, S. 2002. Behaviour of cytokinee levels in serum and peritoneal fluid of women with endometriosis. Gynecol Obstet Invest, 54, 82-87.

Prabowo, R.P., 2005. Endometriosis. In: Wiknjosastro, H., Saifuddin, A.B., and Rachimhadhi, T., Ilmu Kandungan. Jakarta. Yayasan Bina Pustaka Sarwono Prawirohardho: 314-327

Punnonen R, Klemi PJ, Nikkanen V, 1980. Postmenopausal endometriosis, Eur J Obstet Gynecol Reprod Biol 11:195.

Rafiei, A., Hajilooi, M., Shakib, R.J., et al. 2006. Association between the Phe206Leu polymorphism of L-selectin and brucellosis. J Med Microbiol. 55(5):511-516

Ratner BD. Biomaterials science : an introduction to materials in medicine. 2nd ed. Amsterdam ; Boston: Elsevier Academic Press, 2004

Reese KA, Reddy S, Rock JA, 1996. Endometriosis in an adolescent population: the Emory experience, J Pediatr Adolesc Gynecol 9:125.

Rier S, Foster WG, 2003. Environmental dioxins and endometriosis, Seminars Reprod Med 21:145.

Ripps BA, Martin DC, 1992. Correlation of focal pelvic tenderness with implant dimension and stage of endometriosis, J Reprod Med 37:620.

Rosen SD, 2004. Ligands for L-Selectin Homing, Inflammation and Beyond. Annu Rev Immunol. 22:129-156.

Russell, A., Cunninghame, G.D.S., Chadha, S., Roberton, C., Fernandez-Hart, T., Griffiths, B., et al. 2005. No association between E- and L-selectin genes and SLE: soluble L-selectin levels do correlate with genotype and a subset in SLE. Genes Immun. 6(5):422-429

Sangi-Haghpeykar H, Poindexter III AN, 1995. Epidemiology of endometriosis among parous women, Obstet Gynecol 85:983

Saputra I, Siregar HS, et al., 2014. Perbedaan kadar IL-6 pada wanita pendertia endometriosis dan wanita non endometriosis. Universitas Sumatera Utara. Medan.

Sembiring M, Siregar Hs, 2014. Ekspresi Matriks Metalloproteinase 9 Jaringan Endometriosis Dengan Jaringan Normal. Universitas Sumatera Utara. Medan.

Sharpe KL, Zimmer RL, Khan RS, et al. 1992. Proliferative and morphogenic changes induced by the coculture of rat uterine and peritoneal cells: a cell culture model for endometriosis. Fertil Steril;58: 1220-1229.

Sillem M, Prifti S, Monga B, et al. 1999. Integrin mediated adhesion of uterine endometrial cells from endometriosis patients to extracellular matrix proteins is enhanced by TNFalpha and IL-1. Eur J Obstet Gynecol;87:123-127.

Simoens, S., Hummelshoj, L., and D'Hooghe, T., 2007. Endometriosis: cost estimates and methodological perspective. Hum Reprod Update.13(4): 395-404

Spaczynski RZ, Duleba AJ, 2003. Diagnosis of endometriosis, Seminars Reprod Med 21:193.

Sperandio, M., and Ley, K., 2005. The Physiology and Pathophysiology of P-selectin. University of Heidelberg. Germany. Mod. Asp Immunobiol. 15 : 24-26

Stavarachi, M., Apostol, P., Cimponeriu, D., Toma, M., Butoianu, N., and Gavrila, L., 2009. Possible association between L-selectine gene P213S polymorphism and respiratory complications of chidhood spinal muscular atrophy patients. Rom Biotechnol Lett. 14(1): 4119-4122

Strathy, J.H., Molgaard, C.A., Coulam, C.B., and Melton, L.J., 1982. Endometriosis and infertility: a laparoscopic study of endometriosis among fertile and infertile women. Fertil Steril. 38(6): 667-672

Stratton, M. R. and Rahman, N. 008. The emerging landscape of breast cancer susceptibility. Nat Genet, 40, 17-22.

Sundqvist, J., 2011. Pathophysiological factors and genetic association in endometriosis. Stockholm. Karolinska Institutet.

Taylor, R.N., Ryan, I.P., Moore, E.S., Hornung, D., Shifren, J.L., and Tseng, J.F., 1997. Angiogenesis and macrophage activation in endometriosis. Ann N Y Acad Sci. 828:194–207

Tempfer, C.B., Simoni, M., Destenaves, B., and Fauser B.C., 2009. Functional genetic polymorphism and female reproductive disorders: Part II-endometriosis. Hum Reprod Update. 15(1): 97-118

Thiruchelvam U, Dransfield I, Saunders PT, Critchley HO. 2013. The importance of the macrophage within the human endometrium. J Leukoc Biol. 93(2):217-25.

Togashi K, Nishimura K, Kimura I, Tsuda Y, Yamashita K, Shibata T, Nakano Y, Konishi J, Konishi I, Mori T, 1991. Endometrial cysts: diagnosis with MR imaging, Radiology 180:73.

Tran, L.V., Tokushige, N., Berbic, M., Markham, R., and Fraser, I.S., 2009. Macrophages and nerve fibres in peritoneal endometriosis. Hum Reprod. 24(4): 835–841

Tsung, K., Dolan, J.P., Tsung, Y.L., Norton, J.A., 2002. Macrophages as effector cells in interleukin 12-induced T cell-dependent tumor rejection. Cancer Res. 62(17): 5069-5075

Valentine, J.E., 2003. Macrophage Involvement In The Remodelling Of An Extracelluler Matrix Scaffold. B.S. in Materials Science and Engineering, University of Florida: 11-16

Valesco I, Rueda J, Acien P. 2006. Aromatase expression in endometriotic tissues and cell cultures of patients with endometriosis. Molecular Human Reproduction.12:377-381

Verkauf, B.S., 1987. Incidence, symptoms, and signs of endometriosis in infertile and infertile. J Fla Med Assoc. 74(9): 671-675

Wei, Y.,Lan, Y., Meng, L., and Nong, L., 2011. The association of L-selectin polymorphisms with L-selectin serum levels and risk of ischemic stroke. Journal of Thrombosis and Thrombolysis. 32(1): 110-115

Wynn TA, Barron L. 2010. Macrophages: master regulators of inflammation and fibrosis. Semin Liver Dis. 30(3):245-57.

Zeitoun K, Takayama K, Sasano H, Suzuki T, Moghrabi N, Andersson S, Johns A, Meng L, Putman M, Carr B, Bulun SE, 1998. Deficient 17beta-hydroxysteroid dehydrogenase type 2 expression in endometriosis: failure to metabolize 17beta-estradiol, J Clin Endocrinol Metab 83:4474.

Zhang R, Wild RA, Ojago JM. 1993. Effect of tumor necrosis factor-alpha on adhesion of human endometrial stromal cells to peritoneal mesothelial cells: an in vitro system. Fertil Steril;59:1196-1201.

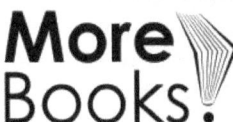
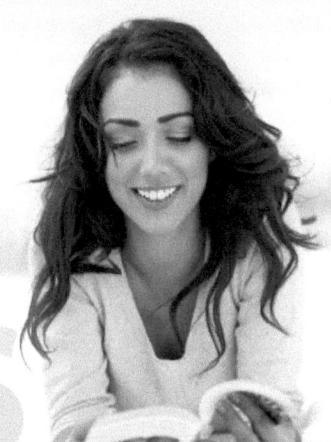

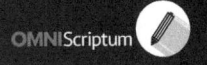

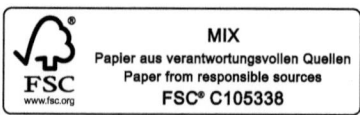